Two-Faced

Confessions of

a Soap Opera

Make-Up Artist

Two-Faced

Confessions of a Soap Opera Make-Up Artist

Timothy Alan

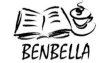

BENBELLA

BenBella Books
6440 N. Central Expressway,
Suite 617
Dallas, TX 75206

BENBELLA

BenBella Books
6440 N. Central Expressway, Suite 617, Dallas, TX 75206
www.benbellabooks.com
Send feedback to feedback@benbellabooks.com

Printed in China
10 9 8 7 6 5 4 3 2 1

Library of Congress Cataloging-in-Publication Data

Alan, Timothy.
  Two-faced : makeup secrets of the soap stars/ by Timothy Alan.

    p. cm.
  ISBN 1-932100-42-3
  1. Beauty, Personal. 2. Cosmetics. 3. Women—Health and hygiene. 4. Television actors and actresses—Health and hygiene. 5. Television makeup. I. Title.

  RA778.A43675 2005
  646.7'042—dc22
            2005007647

Cover design by Lori Casciano, Creativedge Design, Inc.
Text design and composition by Lori Casciano, Creativedge Design, Inc.

Distributed by Independent Publishers Group
To order call (800) 888-4741
www.ipgbook.com

For special sales contact Laura Watkins at laura@benbellabooks.com

This book is dedicated to all of the women who have inspired

me—not only the ones who have allowed me to turn their skin

into a canvas and call it a career but also the ones I have never met ...

the ones who are not on television ...

the ones who sometimes forget when describing themselves

to tack onto the word "ordinary" the word "extra."

I hope this book gives each of you a new appreciation of your

faces—both of them.

Many (Many, Many, Many!) Thanks

If what they say is true, and it takes a village to raise a child, then lemme tell you—it takes almost an entire *country* to complete a book like this!

I'm kidding (but only a little bit).

This book has my name slapped on it, and God knows, at times it's felt like my life's work, but (despite what pictures of me may suggest) my head is not so large that I have any delusions that it would have been possible without the support, guidance and inspiration of a large group of family, friends and colleagues. Foremost among them are the following, to whom I owe a debt of gratitude I'll never be able to repay:

ACKNOWLEDGEMENTS

David Barnum ... What's left to say after 18 years together? Thanks for making this an amazing life.

Patti Small, my sister ... I've changed your diapers, and over the years, watched you change yourself a hundred times. You're an amazing woman now, and I know that when Mom checks up on us, she looks upon you the same way I do—with awe.

My extended family … You have built the character that I have become (or, as the wiseacres among you would put it, you have created this monster!). Thanks for all the laughter and tears and especially for your most precious gift—time.

The ladies who volunteered their rare spare moments, not to mention their faces, to me and to Gilda's Club—some of you without even knowing me ... May the kindness and beauty you rained down upon me mark all the rest of your days. Your generosity of spirit will not be forgotten.

My photographers, Robert Milazzo and Greg Weiner, and last but certainly not least, Alex Kroké ... Guys, your friendship and loyalty are surpassed only by your talent and sweet nature. Without you, I am nothing.

My sketch artist, Age ... Your talent is, no pun intended, timeless. Thanks for so beautifully "penciling me in."

Karen Ross, my PR whiz ... Your abandon and blind faith are so amazing to me that I'm still trying to let go! Ha ha.

All the personal and soap PR reps who juggled time zones and shooting schedules to help me show their clients to my make-up chair ... You went above and beyond time and again, and the results of your Herculean efforts speak for themselves.

Glenn at BenBella Books, my new extended family … Thanks for "adopting" me by optioning this book on its merits and letting me fly. I really appreciate your patience as well as your respect, and I hope that in the end, I earned both and did you proud.

Lori Casciano and the team at Creativedge Design Inc. … Between your baby (literal) and mine (figurative), I didn't know how we'd ever get this all scheduled and done, but wonder of wonders, we did—which, I believe, makes you a wonder of wonders. Your artistic ability is a gift, and your energy, infectious; both of these qualities constantly reminded me that I made the right choice. (And congrats again on your baby ... Ethan is almost as pretty as my baby. Ha ha!)

All of the soap magazines, past and present, for giving me a chance to explore my art form and play with so many great teams over the years.

Finally, I've got to give a shout out to Mimi Torchin, my friends at ABC and all of my Red Bank pals and clients who have supported me financially as well as emotionally. It is because of you all that I am sitting, ahem, pretty.

Thank you!

Timothy Alan

Table of Contents

FOREWORD:

Beauty Call

If there is any force on Earth that elicits a more powerful emotional response than beauty, it can only be love. But while love often strikes as swiftly and as shockingly as lightning, random and unpredictable—and is often as ephemeral—beauty is everywhere, in both nature's magnificent wonders and man's artistic outpourings. From a single feather on a tiny bird to the monumental crashing of waves on a windswept beach, nature's bounty remains timelessly beautiful and, as more of the natural world is destroyed, precious. But human potential for creating or enhancing beauty is endless, and often equally moving.

Beauty is an ineffable quality that affects each of us differently. It can be recognized but can't be defined or pigeonholed. It can't be regulated or dictated, though many political regimes and artistic schools have tried. And if ever a cliché was true, it's that beauty is in the eye of the beholder.

It's a fascinating conundrum that what's beautiful to one person can be an eyesore to another. Consequently, when it comes to standards of personal beauty, one must be true only to oneself, working with the beauty within and without, and avoiding the impossible and ultimately self-defeating pursuit of an externally imposed standard. We are bombarded daily with images of implied perfection on television, in magazines and on the movie screen. Women literally starve themselves to turn perfect, lovely and curvaceous size 8 or 10 bodies into an unnatural and unappealing size 2 or 4. God forbid you should be a size 12 or 14! Undoubtedly, the Hollywood movie and TV studios of today would have put Marilyn Monroe on a diet! In comedian Margaret Cho's hilarious but often painful and personal show, *I'm the One That I Want*, she recounts how she was forced to lose so much weight for her television series that in the process, she also lost her self-esteem and her health. When the show failed, she nearly lost her life, spiraling downward into a world of depression, drugs and alcohol. As if a little fat kept her from being funny, cute, intelligent and unique—the qualities that attracted the network to her in the first place! Men work out until their muscles seem to burst in the pursuit of six-pack abs and the hard, rippled bodies of a Hercules. Both men and women turn workouts into unhealthy obsessions. In the entertainment business in particular, facial plastic surgery for women and men was once relatively rare but is now an everyday practice. On mornings when I've had a bad night's sleep,

You don't have to look like a soap star to be beautiful.

the idea even crosses *my* mind, but fortunately, I always regain my senses by the time I've eaten breakfast! Aging is a part of life, and the tide can be stemmed artificially for only so long before out efforts become grotesque rather than flattering. Better to let nature have her way with us gracefully and with dignity.

And therein lies the rub. We are a society obsessed with youth and the perfection of a youthful beauty. The people who sell everything from toothpaste to tinted contact lenses are interested exclusively, it seems, in this narrowly defined "demographic" (how I hate that word) and have managed to convince us that to be old (older than 49) or imperfect is to be ugly and unwanted. This is humbug at best, immoral at worst. We are all beautiful in our own ways, and what we lack or dislike about out appearance can be enhanced by methods that are natural and healthy. It certainly doesn't hurt (or have to hurt) to look our best. In fact, looking good makes us feel good; it lifts our spirits and our self-esteem.

Ever was it thus. I've been in the business of observing and commenting on soap operas and their stars for more than two

decades, and it's true that, of all the entertainment industries, soaps put the highest premium on beauty. How many times have I heard the phrase "a soap opera look"? This look exists and refers to that exact, idealized, youthful perfection that few possess but many aspire to. The soaps have been accused of sacrificing talent for beauty in their young stars, and this too is something that happens, though less often than those who don't watch soaps would think. What's unfair, however, is that most people do not understand that soaps really make room for all kinds of looks, all ages of beauty, because more than any other genre, daytime drama values its veterans.

When I was founding editor in chief of *Soap Opera Weekly*, the look of my magazine was extremely important to me. Our photography had to be exceptional because we owed it to the stars to make them look their best and to the readers to give them the highest quality art we could. I think anyone who read the magazine during my tenure will agree that our photography was superb. That's because, along with my exceptional photo editor, we employed the best photographers, used the most skilled make-up artists and, rather than just going for a pretty picture, tried to capture something of the internal essence of our subjects. Yes, we wanted them to look "handsome" or "beautiful," but we also wanted to reveal something of their inner beauty and nature.

One of my greatest delights in running *Soap Opera Weekly* was choosing every photo for every major layout for every issue. My photo editor would do an initial edit, and I would then pore over the slides, finding the most interesting images to simultaneously illustrate the story and illuminate the actor. One of the things I always loved about the shoots for which Timothy Alan did the make-up and hair was that the actor always ended up looking completely like him or herself, only better! This was the exact look we wanted: enhancement, not disguise! Tim knows precisely how to achieve this natural but augmented and refined look. Believe me, this isn't something every make-up artist can do. It's a rare gift as well as an art. For daytime drama, the best make-up creates the illusion—under bright, unforgiving lighting—that an actor or actress' good looks are God-given

and unembellished. I think this kind of subtle make-up, while less dramatic and ostentatious, is every bit as much of an art form.

In this book, Tim will show you, step by step, how you can achieve the same results at home, with a minimum of fuss and a maximum of results. His goal is to help you make the most of your own assets, to let you look like you, only better! In the interviews that accompany the photos, several of your favorite stars of various ages will share with you their personal beauty secrets, diet regimens and philosophies of living a "beautiful life." In addition to learning a treasure trove of interesting information about these actresses as well as their valuable beauty tips, you'll hopefully gain some insights into your own feelings about yourself. But never forget: There are all kinds of beauty in the world. You don't have to look like a soap star to be beautiful. You are all beautiful already. But if it's something you'd like to do—and presumably, it's one of the reasons you've bought this book—by the time you finish *Two-Faced: Confessions of a Soap Opera Make-Up Artist*, you will know how to recreate the look of your favorite actress. Have fun,

because at its best, that's another thing make-up should be.

Mimi Torchin

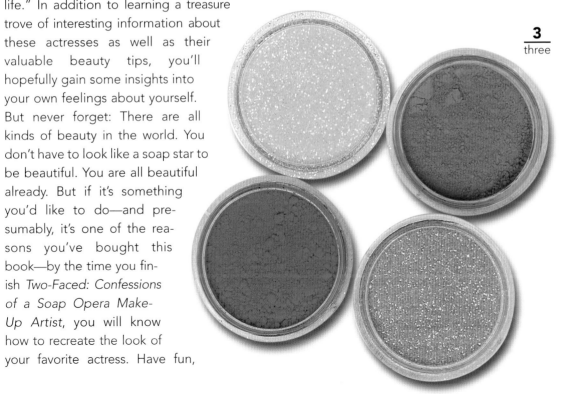

PREFACE:
Here's Lookin' at You

Were you ever a kid with stars in your eyes? I was. And since I come from a military family with a background in electrical engineering, really that was the height of impracticality. Seriously—can you imagine the reaction I got when one night at the dinner table I told my mother that I wanted to grow up to be either a make-up artist or a mortician? First, there was a dramatic pause. Then, creeped out, she said, "Nobody in our family works with the dead." Plan B was equally well received. My brother threw open the front door and asked, "See any stars out there?" I wanted to reply, "No, but when I *do* start working with beautiful actresses every day, you can bet I won't be introducing them to *you*!" Instead, I asked my mother to pass the mashed potatoes.

Luckily, my Aunt Kathy baby-sat me with great frequency. A pageant regular, she'd often arrive with her hair rolled in beer cans and her make-up in a round box with a snappy little handle. To this day, she insists that, as my first muse, she is owed a big commission. (Let's just see how the book does first, okay, Auntie?) She would paint her face endlessly and at times, I'd swear Michelangelo's work on the Sistine Chapel didn't take as long. Then she'd surround her ratted hair with a cloud of spray that only I could walk on. I loved every bit of it. To me, it was pure and honest and quite beautiful—and those memories remain among my fondest. Heck, if it weren't for the stars in *her* eyes, the ones in my own might well have been dimmed or snuffed out altogether. (Okay, Aunt Kathy, you'll get your commission.)

After my mother passed away, long after I had quit slipping make-up palettes into

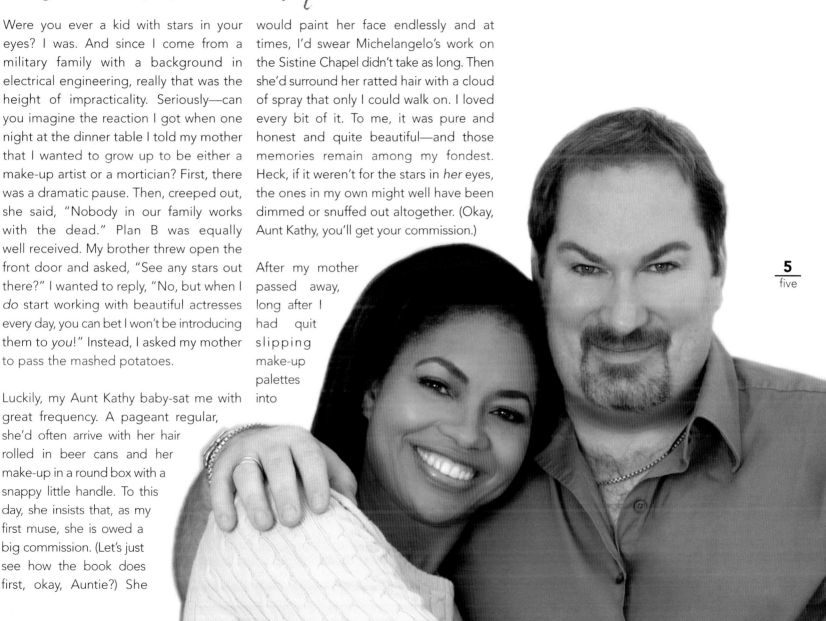

her grocery cart, I moved almost immediately to New York. I can still remember the best piece of advice she ever gave me, though: Be careful what you choose as your career; what you do for a living could wind up being your life's work. Boy, was she ever right. A series of department-store make-up counter jobs led to my first freelance assignments—and an embarrassing episode involving myself, some amateur Polaroids and some extremely kind *Cosmo* editors who told me to get a book together and come back. I soon got so busy that I never *did* go back. But then, out of the blue, my phone rang. It was a photographer by the name of Robert Milazzo asking if I was free for a shoot. It wasn't a cover or anything like that … it was even better! The subject of the session was Helen Gurley Brown, sitting for her last portrait as editor in chief of *Cosmo*. Whoa. It's pretty cool when everything falls into place, but it's even cooler when it doesn't, and the way you rearrange things allows fate to sneak in through an open window.

Now, all these years later—I mean, all these years of *my* life later, but if you've gotten bored, you may feel like it's years later in *your* life as well—we arrive at this book, a labor of love. Way back when I was being mocked over meatloaf and creamed corn by my family, I never would have imagined that the stars I once pictured would pale in comparison to the stars with whom I'd actually collaborate. But strange and wonderful things happen when you dare to dream—the strangest and most wonderful of all being that occasionally dreams do come true. For me, that meant one thing leading to another and another until finally I had practiced my trade on most of daytime television's grande dames, from *All My Children*'s Susan Lucci to *Guiding Light*'s Kim Zimmer.

At this point, I can just hear you saying, "Yes, yes, what a fascinating life you've led. Big whoop—did you have to write a book about it? And even if you did, why do I have to read it?"

The first question is easy. In the more than two decades since I began working with soap actresses, I have marveled at how two-faced they really are—and not in a double-talking, hair-pulling kind of way, either. Day after day, these women work their tails off, being kidnapped and shot at, tried and convicted, seduced and dropped like hot potatoes. And in their free time—obviously a relative term in their world—they are devoted wives and doting moms, savvy businesswomen and dazzling singers. When they say, "I've done it all," they not only mean it, they usually mean that they did it on their

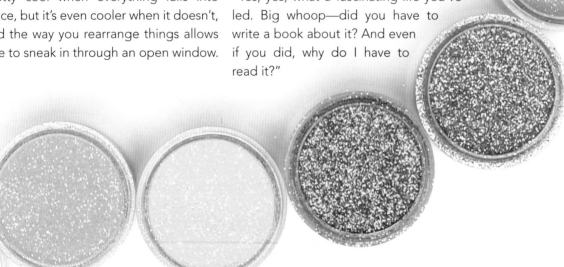

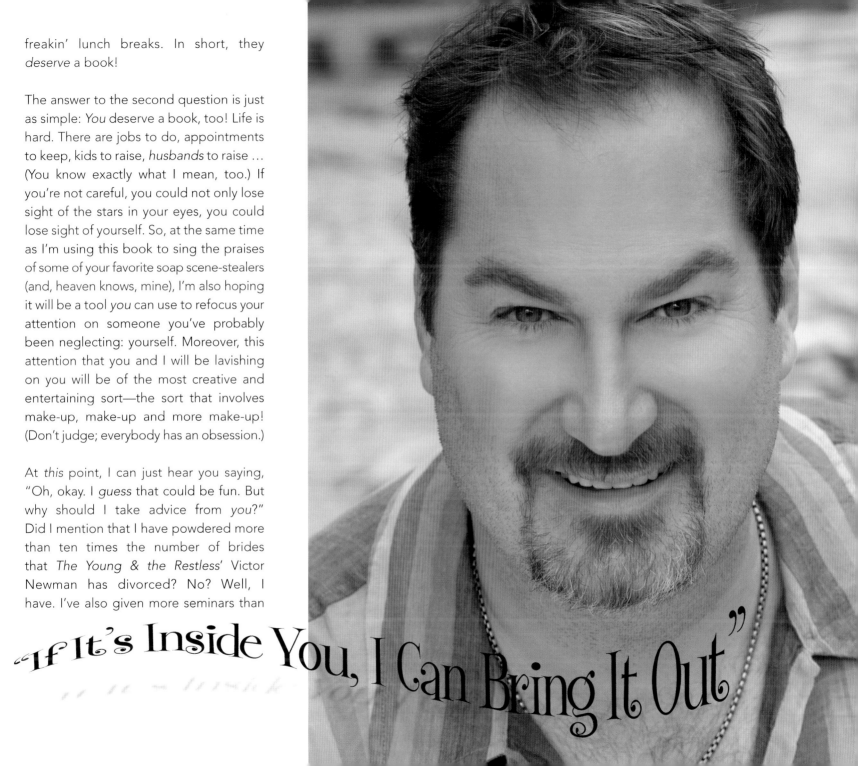

freakin' lunch breaks. In short, they *deserve* a book!

The answer to the second question is just as simple: *You* deserve a book, too! Life is hard. There are jobs to do, appointments to keep, kids to raise, *husbands* to raise … (You know exactly what I mean, too.) If you're not careful, you could not only lose sight of the stars in your eyes, you could lose sight of yourself. So, at the same time as I'm using this book to sing the praises of some of your favorite soap scene-stealers (and, heaven knows, mine), I'm also hoping it will be a tool *you* can use to refocus your attention on someone you've probably been neglecting: yourself. Moreover, this attention that you and I will be lavishing on you will be of the most creative and entertaining sort—the sort that involves make-up, make-up and more make-up! (Don't judge; everybody has an obsession.)

At *this* point, I can just hear you saying, "Oh, okay. I *guess* that could be fun. But why should I take advice from *you*?" Did I mention that I have powdered more than ten times the number of brides that *The Young & the Restless*' Victor Newman has divorced? No? Well, I have. I've also given more seminars than

"If It's Inside You, I Can Bring It Out"

...you and only you truly own your beauty.

General Hospital's Carly Corinthos has given kisses, and I've made more soap actresses blush than incorrigible leading men who insist on doing love scenes in their thongs. I rattle off this list of dubious achievements not to toot my own horn (although it *is* kind of fun; you should try it sometime) but to assure you that when I say I know what I'm talking about, boy do I ever!

Plus, trust is going to be very important in the relationship that we are about to establish. I know that not everyone has nerves of steel. In my travels, I've met many, many women who look at a make-up kit like it's a Pandora's box. They—and maybe you—are afraid that if they make one false move, they'll be scarred for life. Relax; that ain't the way it works. This stuff washes off. Unlike a bad haircut or an ex with delusions of possibility, a messy make-up job is easily dispatched. Furthermore, if you use your head—and avail yourself of the wealth of knowledge in my pea brain—no one will ever guess that there was a time when you weren't applying your cosmetics like a whiz.

Feel better now? I thought you might. Bet the stars in your eyes have even begun twinkling anew.

But wait, wait, wait! Don't go skipping ahead to the chapters on eyebrow-plucking and lip-lining just yet.

First, I want to give you the lowdown on my approach to make-up. If you get to know this little bit about me now, you'll have a good chuckle later every time you roll your eyes and say, "Oh, that's just Tim!"

Now then, my overall make-up theory is the same as Britney Spears' is (only she applies her theory to clothing rather than cosmetics): Less is more. If you need an extra coat of mascara on your eyelashes, odds are that no one will notice unless he is right in your face (and, honey, once you've got a guy *that* close, he ought to have better things to do than offer up a critique). On the other hand, if you err on the side of excess, people will be able to see your mistake (and snicker at it) a block away. So there you have it—that's the entire basis of the book you now have in your hands. (Keep flipping pages, though; the devil's in the details, and the pictures sure are purdy.)

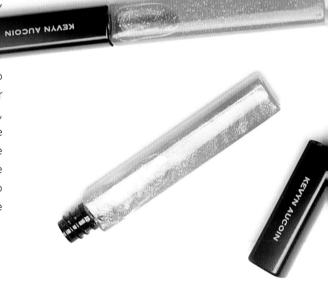

In the chapters that follow, you will read about a million of my dire warnings and brilliant suggestions, all meant to insure that you put your best face forward. But as you study them (and I know you will … um, won't you?), remember that you and only you truly own your beauty. So don't let me, some chick behind the make-up counter or anybody else try to convince you that you should put on a face that would be … well, a put-on. You are the judge and jury when it comes to what looks and feels right on you. The rest of us? We're just the peanut gallery, full of opinions, all of which are inconsequential if they differ from your own.

Furthermore, as you look at the photos in this book—or in any magazine—remember that they have been touched up. What you see in print is not necessarily what you get in person—and that's okay. These minor works of art, just like the most highfalutin ads you could conceivably come across, are fiction—just like the stories on *Days of Our Lives* and *General Hospital*. They are reflections of a heightened reality. And if you hold yourself up to those precise, carefully calculated standards, you will always fall short. You are not Erica Kane, nor are you Olivia Spaulding or Theresa Lopez Fitzgerald. You are who you are—and that's different, yeah, but it's no less beautiful. So—and I know this may be hard, but try anyway, don't compare yourself to characters. Don't compare yourself at all.

What sets you apart from everybody else here in the real world—including the real women in this book—is what is on the inside. That's a cliché, I know, but clichés are often clichés because they are true. (Hello?! That's why they *become* clichés.) If it isn't the soul that sets us all apart from one another, in equally impressive ways, then I'm at a loss, because it seems to me that everything on the outside fades (or packs on pounds or gets splotchy or … you get the picture). With make-up, we are just adding plumage to the rare bird that you already are. See? It's just like you tried to tell your self-absorbed college boyfriend with the skateboard: In this case, it *is* all about you.

That's why, in the next eight chapters, we're going to take an inside-out approach to you and your marvelous mug: The beauty's already in you; we just need to bring it (all together now) *out*. (We will, too, kiddo.) Maybe all that means is that you need a pep talk. Perhaps it will require that your eyebrows be tweezed with a weed whacker. But whatever it takes, we'll do it. Then, voila! You'll feel good. And if you feel good, you'll look better. (It's a circle, but not the vicious kind.) And if you feel crummy, fake it; you might fool yourself, and you'll certainly convince others to buy into the illusion, just the way

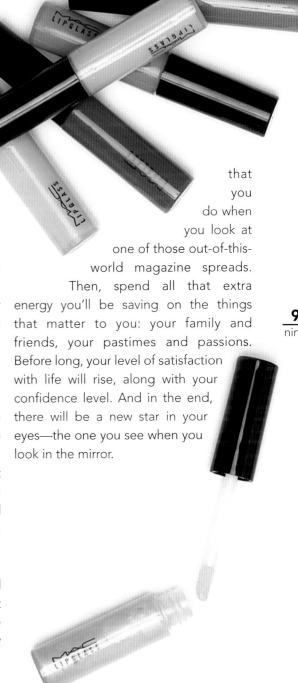

that you do when you look at one of those out-of-this-world magazine spreads. Then, spend all that extra energy you'll be saving on the things that matter to you: your family and friends, your pastimes and passions. Before long, your level of satisfaction with life will rise, along with your confidence level. And in the end, there will be a new star in your eyes—the one you see when you look in the mirror.

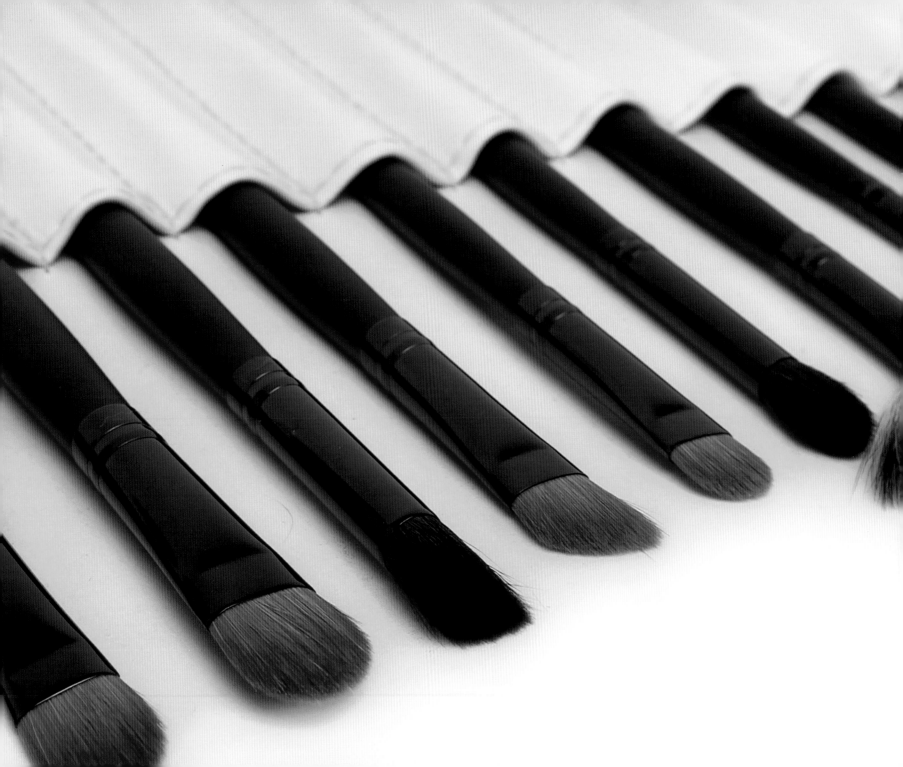

CHAPTER 1:

Tool Time

"The right tool for the right job." That's what my father always told me. Well, that and, "Get a haircut, kid; you ain't Ringo Starr." But the point he *really* wanted to make, and make stick, was the one about the tools. Naturally, as a budding make-up artist, I thought I had about as much use for that old adage as a hairdresser does for a drill. Dad was mortified, of course—not only did Junior prefer applying foundation to laying it, but his sage advice was destined to fall on deaf ears. Little did we know ... Years later—and don't bother asking me how many; I'm only revealing *beauty* secrets here—I realized that my father was absolutely right. (When he reads this, I suspect—nay, hope—that he will say, "I told you so." He deserves a moment of vindication.) I still expect orange juice and vodka when I ask for a screwdriver, and think that if a stud finder isn't a dating service, it should be, but I have also come to see that, regardless of your trade, it pays to know your tools. Whether your line of work takes you to Ace Hardware's monkey-wrench department or the cosmetics counter at Bergdorf-Goodman, the principle is the same.

Lucky for me, I am well versed in my tools. Lucky for you, these are the same implements that you will need to transform yourself from plain Jane to plumb amazing.

When women ask me which doodads and thingamabobs to purchase, I always paraphrase Tina Turner: "Simply the best," I reply. I'm not being flip, either. (I mean, don't get me wrong: I can be more flip than a *That Girl!* hairdo, but a discussion of cosmetic accoutrements is no place for sarcasm.) Think about it: The better the tool, the better it will work and the longer it will last. See? It's not rocket science. Select your applicators with great enough care, and you may find yourself with a purseful of new best friends who will neither borrow money nor steal your boyfriend.

In my collection—or, as I prefer to call it, "my arsenal," since my weapons of choice are ever-ready for "complective" combat—I have about 200 brushes, of which I generally use from 24 to 48 make-up brushes until they finally crumble and force me to play "Taps" for them. As a comparably normal human being, chances are you won't need nearly that many of anything—that is, unless you are hoping to establish a reputation for yourself as the Imelda Marcos of make-up. However, if you stock up selectively, and take care of your arsenal as I do, it will always take care of you.

So, what will you actually need? May I suggest a few key components of my travel pack—if you will, a make-up maven's top 10 totes?

1. A toothbrush, preferably new or at least sterilized and no longer being used to whitewash your choppers. (Technically, i suppose you don't have to buy a toothbrush exclusively for make-up application. But if you don't... well, not to put too fine a point on it or anything, but ew!) This, you will use to tame your eyebrows and blend in your brow shading. Works like a charm. And leaves your brows feeling unusually minty-fresh!

2. A pocket mirror. i use mine to allow my clients to see extreme close-ups of themselves (and also to reassure myself that they aren't vampires). You will more likely use yours to double-check that your handiwork was, in fact, handy.

3. A small pair of scissors. Remember those brows we talked about taming? Consider this your whip and your chair. Scissors are perfect for trimming brows that have become too long. They also help to keep you from resembling Andy Rooney between visits to your brow landscaper.

4. An eyelash curler. Everybody needs one of these, period. Except for those of you who don't. And by "those of you who don't," i obviously mean "those of you who every other woman in the world hates with a fiery passion."

5. Q-Tips. Yes, they're not just for de-waxing your ears anymore. They're also great for quick clean-ups and subtle blending. Not all Q-Tips are created equal, either: The best of the bunch are the fiber-free variety with the wooden handles. Whenever i find them, i buy in bulk. i do the same thing with Peeps, but that's another story—

6. Tweezers. C'mon! You didn't think that that stray hair was going to just vanish for you out of pity, did you? And those false eyelashes ... how are they supposed to know when it's time to call it a night? Face it—you're going to need tweezers.

7. Sponges. No "Seinfeld" jokes, okay? You are all sponge-worthy. That said, go for the latex-free triangle kind—there's virtually no area into which they won't fit.

8. A pencil sharpener, because there's no point in trying to apply lip liner with a dull pencil. No point ... get it? Oh, never mind.

9. Brushes, brushes and more brushes! Maybe not 200, but a whole bunch nonetheless. You will need one for powder and one for blush, a lip brush, a bronzing brush, an eyebrow brush (angled, preferably), some (brace yourself for a very technical term) "large fluff" eye brushes for the general eye area, an eyeliner brush for the detail work (the closer to the lashes you get, the trickier the job becomes), a smudger brush, a "medium fluff" brush for blending and finishing, and a "small fluff" brush to dispatch the crease area. You know, on second thought, you actually may need 200 brushes to be pretty. Kidding. (You can get by with 150. Kidding again.)

10. Tissues, because accidents happen. You'll need these puppies to tidy up, to serve as a clean surface on which everything else can rest, and to hand to the weepy lotharios whose hearts you are destined to break when you realize that you can do better.

By and by, you will arrive at your own personal favorites. Trust me—you'll be embarrassed later if right now you try to sound like a mother lioness, saying, "No, I'll love them all equally." There will be some that you can't live without and others you'll forget why you ever bought them in the first place. In the meantime, don't be afraid to ask other women (in particular the ones whose looks you like) what's in their kits. Heaven knows, people are always curious about what's in mine. Heck, every time I've done make-up for a wedding, I've drawn a crowd!

Above all, remember, good tools are better than cheap ones. Armed with any old things, you may be able to get by, but honey, you won't be able to get beautiful! Put together your mini kit with care, slowly and surely, committing to a new addition only when you are sure of its merits. Yes, I know—it's a lot like settling on any

relationship. Choose wisely, and odds are, your kit will outlast … what was his name again?

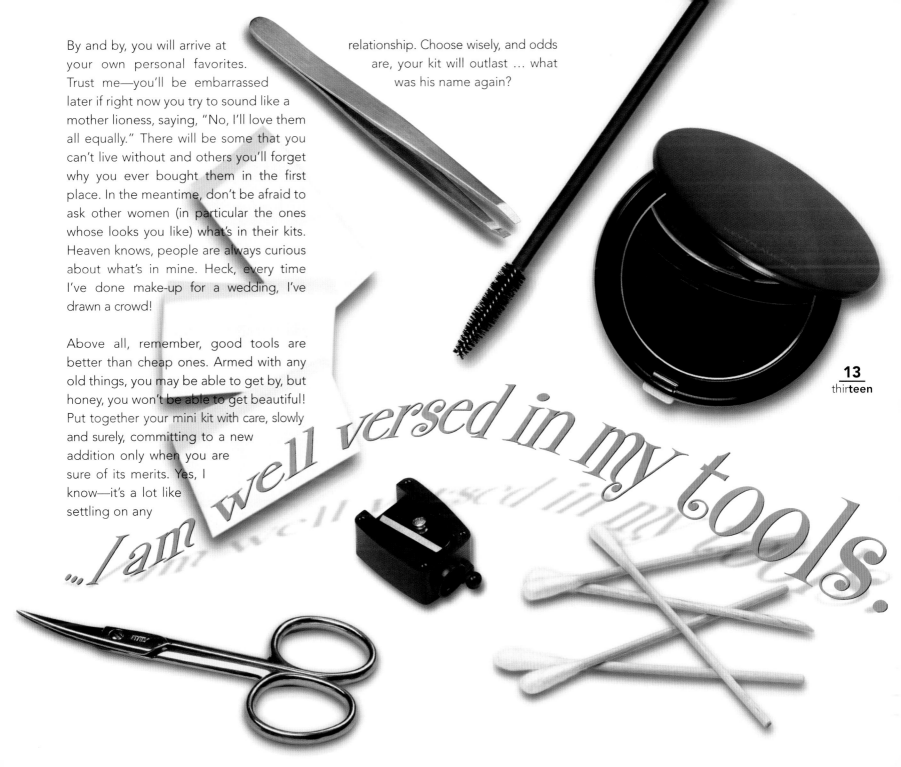

...I am well versed in my tools.

HILLARY B. SMITH

What I love most about Hillary B. Smith is how little she carries herself like a beginner starlet fresh off the turnip truck. Where showbiz is concerned, she's been around the block, so she can tell you where *all* the potholes are! Mind you, she's not *just* a tough cookie—she's sweet, too. But she possesses a self-awareness that is almost intimidating: She knows her strengths and, one suspects, can spot other people's a mile away. No doubt, the Emmy victor came by her wisdom the hard way. Heaven knows she's paid her dues! Soap aficionados have seen her hop from one plum role (Kit McCormick during the final year of *The Doctors*) to another (*As the World Turns*' Margo Hughes after *First Daughter*'s Margaret Colin and before Ellen Dolan), finally settling into the part she was born to play: *One Life to Live*'s Nora Buchanan, the barrister giving the best banter since Hepburn met Tracy. In addition, she's headlined her own sitcom, *Something Wilder*, with Gene Wilder, and struck gold on the silver screen opposite some major movie stars (tops on the list: Sandra Bullock in *Love Potion No. 9* and J.Lo in *Maid in Manhattan*). Someone whom I can only assume is her doppelganger—because really, where would the real McCoy find the time?—is also raising two children with her husband, Phillip "Nip" Smith. Want to know how comfortable in her own skin is this shrewd operator?

Read on…

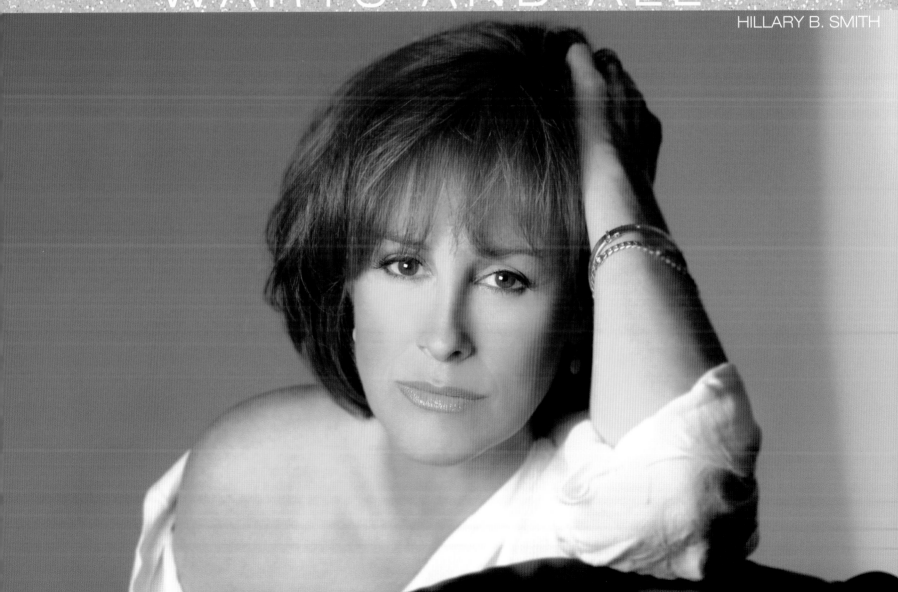

"I OWN MY OWN BEAUTY,
WARTS AND ALL"

HILLARY B. SMITH

What is beauty to you?
Inner beauty is the best kind of beauty.

Funny, that's exactly the message I want people to take away from this book! (*Aside to Hillary*) The check's in the mail. (*Out loud*) I jest! Of course I jest! So, tell me, where beauty is concerned, what, if anything, do you have to hide?
Nothing. I own my beauty, warts and all.

For the record, readers, Hillary actually has no warts whatsoever. On an unrelated topic, what's your favorite pick-me-up?
Well, a good martini is a perfect relaxant.

(*Hiccups*) No kidding. Who taught you about the ins and outs of beauty?
I learned the most from my mother.

It never ceases to amaze me how many women say that—I did, too, and my mother never wore make-up. She was a classic beauty. So do you hate any beauty products—and please, be nice; this is a make-up book, after all!
(*Laughs*) Eyelash curler. What the hell?! Ouch!

What are you most proud of?
My children. Without a doubt.

I have a feeling they're pretty proud of you, too. Which of your soap storylines was the most fun for you?
The rape trial [in which *OLTL*'s Nora sold out her own client upon realizing that he was guilty of the crime].

That *was* intense. Who's been your favorite leading man?
Gene Wilder [my husband on the sitcom *Something Wilder*].

Ah, how perfect that this book is helping Gilda's Club [which was begun in honor of his late wife Gilda Radner]. Let's have a little fun, okay? Tell me the guy you'd really like to share a steamy scene with!
Hmmmmmm. The mind reels. (*Finally*) George Clooney. He's so funny.

Hmmmmmm. Yes, he's definitely drop-dead funny. Other than the *Out of Sight* DVD, do you have a late-night treat?
Sure do—my husband.

Awwww. That's so sweet. (*Aside to Hillary*) Don't worry; I won't tell George. (*Out loud*) Do you have a philosophy of life?
Yes, I do. "Life's a banquet, and most poor suckers are starving to death. Live, live, live!" The quote is from *Mame*, the movie.

Rosalind Russell—now *there's* a bawdy dame! Speaking of bawdy, what about a guy turns you on?
Hmmmmmmm …

Okay. George Clooney, it is. What beauty advice do you have for the younger set?
You can't buy enhancement … it truly is inside of you.

You're preachin' to the choir now, sister! Hallelujah! What's the best gift you have ever been given?
Life.

May I call you *Mame*?

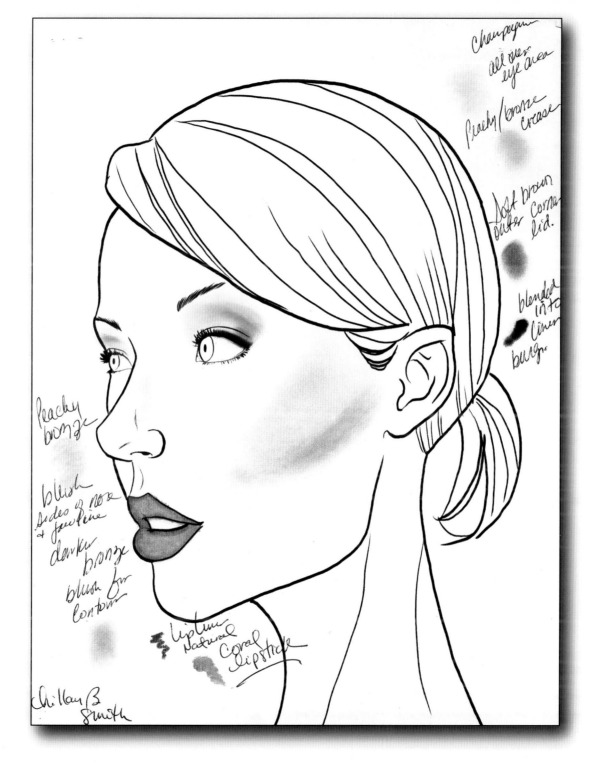

STEPHANIE GATSCHET

I only met Stephanie Gatschet for the first time recently, but when I did, I got the strangest sensation: I felt as if I'd known her all my life. Seriously. She's kind of quiet and quite thoughtful, and has the presence of the quintessential girl next door. Certainly, she made me wish she was the girl next door to *me*. (Memo to self: time to relocate to a nicer neighborhood.) So I have to give *Guiding Light* props for pulling her out of college to play Tammy Winslow. Sure, the tormented teen's mother is a former stripper and her ill-fated adoptive father was a prince/used-car salesman. None of that matters; Tammy remains the sort of sweetheart a boy could know for years before waking up one day to realize he should've been filling her locker with love notes the whole time. Even if you can't tell by looking at Stephanie how unassuming a beauty she is, you probably *can* guess that she's a big softy. Those doe eyes of hers are inevitably drawn to four-legged friends, making her membership in the Humane Society a no-brainer. And if all of this doesn't make you wish you at least *felt* as if you'd known her all your life, read this transcript of our chat; you're gonna.

'DON'T CONFORM TO ANYONE'S STANDARD OF BEAUTY"

STEPHANIE GATSCHET

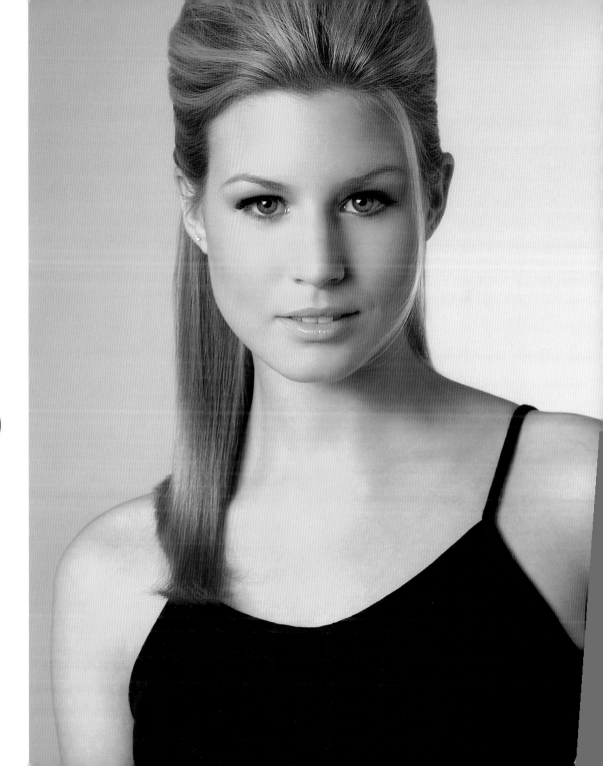

What does beauty mean to you?
Having confidence, feeling good and strong, and having a good heart.

Where beauty is concerned, what do you have to hide, if anything?
I don't hide a thing, but when my butt feels big, I flaunt it.

Me, too—if by "flaunt it," you mean "bury my face in a bag of Oreos." If I were to drop by your place and find you just chilling out, what would you be wearing?
Sweatpants, a t-shirt and knit socks.

Hot! How do you stay in shape?
I live in a fifth-floor walk-up, and I walk my dog, Chichi, anywhere from three to five times a day.

That's why when I lived in the city, I had a cat. When you travel, what are your staples?
Sneakers, hoodies and sundresses.

That reminds me of a funny story. Once, I bought my sister a sundress for a blind date, and … On second thought, I want my sister to let me live. What is your favorite pick-me-up?
Mountain Dew 20 oz., first thing in the morning.

Yeah, coffee is for the faint of heart. What's your favorite piece of clothing?
My ripped-up, low-rise Lucky jeans.

I'll *bet* they're lucky! Do you believe make-up has power?
I *know* make-up has power—my boyfriend is a hunk!

That reminds me of a funny story about my sister's sundress and a blind date … If only she wouldn't kill me! What do you feel is your best feature?
My eyes.

So I see. And your worst?
My worst feature is my butt, but I don't let it get me down.

Who taught you the most about beauty?
My mother. She taught me that beauty is from the inside out.

Lucky for me she didn't write this book first! When do you feel the most beautiful?
At the beach, because it's easy beauty. It's all very natural.

What is the make-up product that you hate the most?
I hate foundation.

Listen to you! That's because you have nothing to hide. Let's play favorites, starting with … your favorite smell.
Geranium.

Taste?
Vanilla.

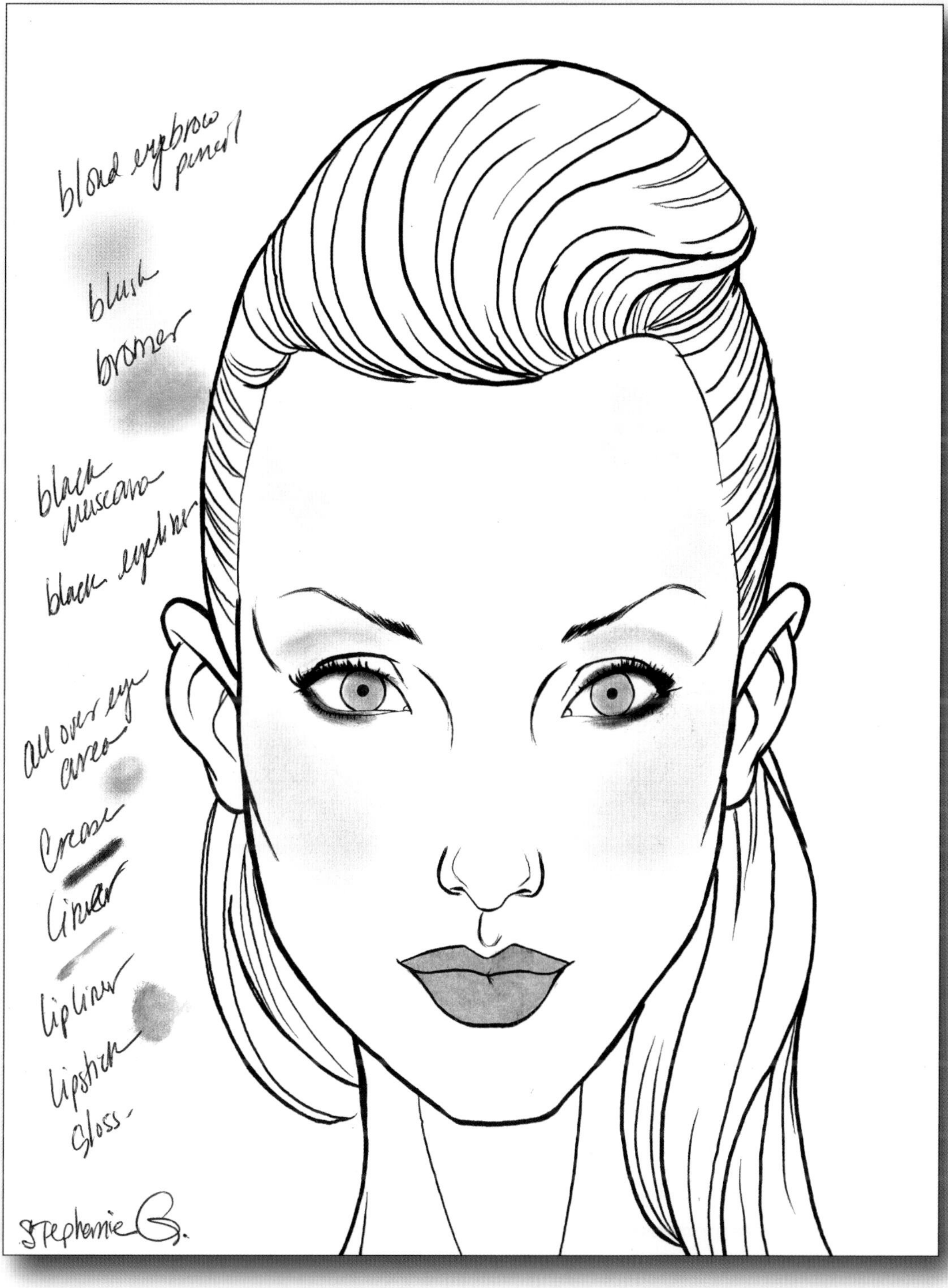

blond eyebrow pencil

blush

bronzer

black mascara

black eyeliner

All over eye area

Crease

Liner

Lip liner

Lipstick
Gloss.

Stephanie B.

Sound?
Nature.

Touch?
My boyfriend's.

Should've seen that one comin'. Sight?
Happy people.

Especially the happy people who are also shiny. What is the hardest lesson you have learned in your 21 years?
I have learned that big change is a part of life.

What do you think is the best age for young girls to start wearing make-up?
Depends on doing what make-up at what age. For example, no mascara on a 4-year-old, but lip gloss on an 8-year-old? Sure.

Have you ever had your make-up done at a department-store cosmetics counter?
Yes. It was great. It was the first time. I knew no better.

What is the most confusing part of the beauty routine to you?
Hair color. I used to do it from a box until Laura Wright (who plays my mom, Cassie, on *Guiding Light*) introduced me to her colorist. He's amazing.

I'll say. I've worked with Laura since she joined the show, and no matter the hairdo she is doing, she always pulls it off with flying colors. What are you most proud of?
Sticking with my goals.

Me, too—like finishing this book! What is the storyline you had the most fun doing?
My favorite was with David Andrew Macdonald (who plays Cassie's brother-in-law and husband, Edmund, on *Guiding Light*). I was supposed to be in love with my uncle. The storyline was kinda creepy, but it was so much fun to do with David.

What's the most beneficial thing that working in daytime has afforded you?
Being able to support myself in New York City.

I remember when I first moved here, that was a very big accomplishment—and as soon as you realize that you're doing it, it's too late to get on the train to go back home! Who is your favorite male co-star?
All of them. They are really *hot*.

You must like doing the romantic storylines, then.
I have only had the one, with David.

Right. Your uncle-kissing plot. So who would you *like* to have a sexy screen moment with?
Danny Cosgrove (who plays Bill).

What has been your favorite pet?
Chichi, my Chihuahua mix.

Getting back to beauty, do you read beauty books?
No, but I'll read this one!

You'd better! Even Chichi gets a shout-out! Do you feel soap stars get the credit they deserve?
Not really. Nobody realizes how hard they work to put on an hour show each day.

Hey, that's reason No. 710 why I'm doing this book. Uncanny! Do have any hidden talents that fans might not know about?
I am a classical pianist.

What was the last book you read?
How to Meditate. I loved it!

Aside from your boyfriend, what is your favorite late-night treat?
Junk food … any kind. Just junk food.

What attracts you most to a guy?
His smile.

And repels you?
Arrogance.

Now we're talkin'! "Don't hate the player, hate the game"? Uh, no, let's go ahead and hate the player.
What do you think is the most important thing for young women to know today about the myth of beauty?
Don't conform to anyone's standard of beauty. Only be the best you can be.

When did you realize the power of being a woman?
At college, when I was living on my own. I was taking care of myself.

What was the happiest day of your life?
Do I have to pick just one? I am so lucky; all
my days are happy.

Let's hear it for that boyfriend!

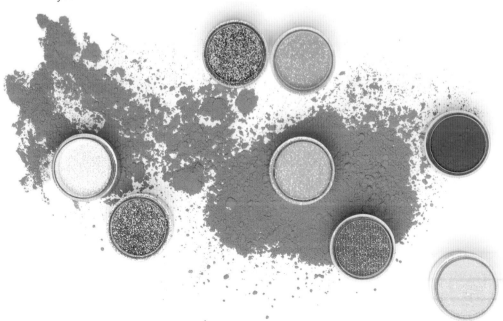

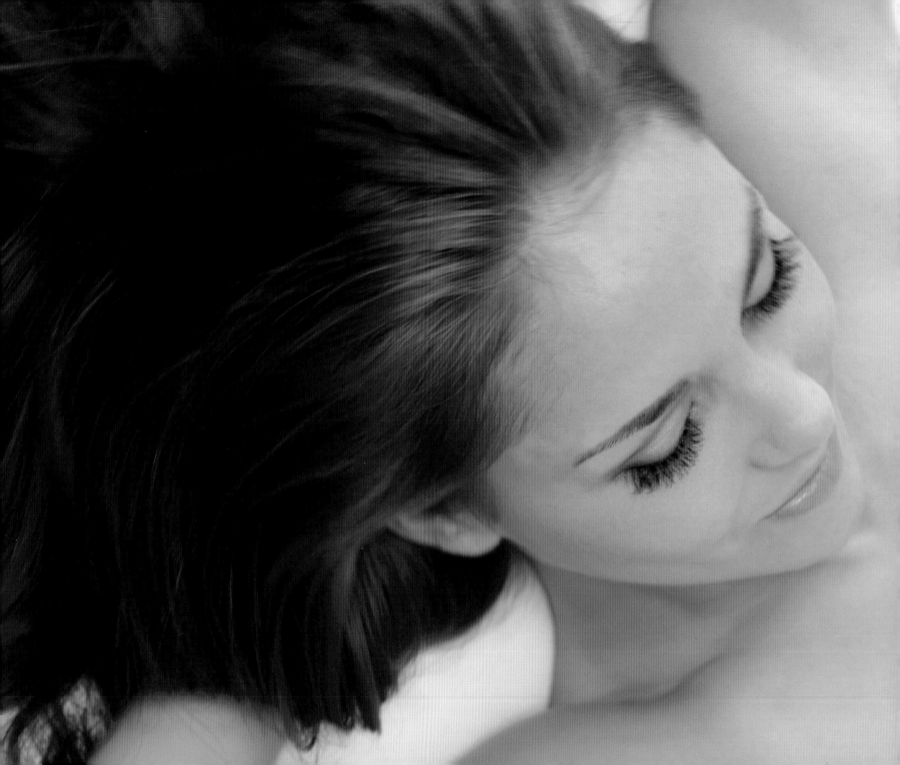

CHAPTER 2:

Saving Face

I know, I know: You're tired of reading about brushes and sponges and everything in between; you want to get to the friggin make-up already.

Not so fast, missy!

Before we start slapping paint on that mug o' yours, we're going to go through a quick tutorial on how to protect it. After all, you can replace a tube of lipstick easily enough, but a new face … that's another story altogether, no matter what *Extreme Makeover* and *The Swan* would have you believe.

Really, this master's class in complexion contains little more than common-sense reminders, so if you find yourself reading along, thinking, "Yeah, yeah, tell me something I *don't* know!" bully for you. Here's your gold star; your mama raised you right (and probably still looks like a million bucks herself). But for those of you who may be startled to learn that nobody's skin glows without their drinking enough water to bloat a camel or who think wearing your make-up to bed is the most fool-proof way to make sure that loverboy is still warming his pillow in the morning, read closely, re-read and, for your own good, take copious notes. Now then, on we go.

1 DIRTY MIND? GOOD. DIRTY FACE? EH, NOT SO MUCH.

No matter how hungover you are, or who you might be expecting to serve you breakfast in bed, you should wash your face morning and night. (Hey, don't whine: At least it's not like brushing your teeth; can you imagine breaking out the Noxzema every time you ate a Triscuit?) Following the cleansing, apply a stabilizing lotion. Sometimes called a toner—or, if I'm around, anti-depressants for your pores—this product removes the balance of cleanser, prepares the skin for moisturizing (because, you know, your skin really hates surprises) and normalizes your skin's pH level.

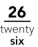

Is this important? Only as important as whether you look fine or freakin' fantastic! In other words, yes. Think about it: If you put make-up on skin that is lacking in moisture or, God forbid, is too oily or dirty, you'll end up resembling your favorite star *after* a bender and not before. Plus, if you keep your skin in tip-top shape, you'll find that you actually need less make-up to achieve that "naturally pretty" look that usually takes so much work. Neat trick, huh? Thought you'd like that.

2 YOU CAN'T GET WET 'N' WILD WITHOUT GETTING WET.

You know those women you always see running around with a gallon jug of water? They've got the right idea. I'll grant you, you've got your work cut out for you, finding clothes that'll go with a clutch purse by Poland Springs. But your skin will thank you, and so will anyone who touches it, if you keep enough H_2O flowing through Y-O-U.

Naturally, you need to hydrate and moisturize your outsides as well as your insides. How much moisturizer you need, and where you need it, is your call. My general rule of thumb is, if it feels dry or tight to the touch, let it pour; if it feels oily, get yourself an oil-control product, and fast, before your complexion starts drawing comparisons to the Exxon-Valdez.

Before we move on, one last point about hydration: The eyes have it, and if they don't, they need it. Jeepers—the area around your peepers has some of the thinnest skin on the body, so it stands to reason that it requires special care. My advice: eye cream in the morning, eye cream in the evening. No questions asked (because if you ask a question, my answer will only be, "You need eye cream in the morning and the evening, dammit!").

You should only apply eye cream to the brow bone and the top of the cheek area. (You should be able to feel the top of the cheekbone at the corner of your eye.) Be careful, though: You don't ever want to get product in your lashes, because from there, it's just one swipe of the hand before it is in your eyes.

3 IF IT AIN'T BROKE…
AW, NUTS!
WHAT IF IT IS BROKE?

Got blemishes? Blotches? Rosacea? Other problems that are too big and bizarre to name (without a degree in dermatology and a translator, anyway)? Consult with a pro. Your skincare specialist will help you come up with the best plan of attack, no matter how gnarly your condition may be. (Self-diagnosis and treatment may actually make matters worse, so, although I'm a big proponent of taking risks, this is one that I can say with great certainty you should pass up!)

These days, there is almost nothing that doctors can't handle—affordably, too. Above all, bear in mind that no matter what your nasty ex says, you are not a snake, therefore you will not have the option of shedding your skin. What you see is what you've got. Treat it well, and it will last you, conveniently enough, a lifetime.

4 HERE COMES THE SUN! QUICK! RUN! HIDE!

Don't let that headline scare you—much. As warm and inviting as it is, the sun can actually do both your face and your heart a lot of good. But it's a little bit like sour-apple martinis—best in moderation. Ignore that advice, about either the sun *or* the martinis, and you'll be sorry. (Don't forget, tomato juice and Tylenol may be able to stop your head from throbbing, but they'll do zilch to keep your damaged skin from scaring the bejesus out of your mirror.)

Mind you, I'm not advocating a life that excludes the great outdoors—c'mon, the outdoors is so cool, it has "great" right there in its name. But I *am* saying that you need to protect yourself. Wear a sunblock. Wear a hat—i.e., the fashion plate's sunblock of choice. Then go nuts—hop on a boat, walk in the park, look for clouds in the shape of your fourth boyfriend's birthmark. Take a few precautions for the sake of your complexion, and the world can be your oyster. Bon appétit!

KNIVES...
THEY'RE NOT JUST
FOR BACKSTABBING ANYMORE.

I have to be honest here … Well, okay, I don't *have* to be, but I think you and I have established a certain rapport at this point, and I wouldn't want to do anything now to shake your faith. My views on plastic surgery are as blurry as a soap heroine's vision after she's been slipped a mind-erasing drug. To me, the "Should I or shouldn't I?" question all depends on the procedure you are considering and, perhaps even more importantly, the reason you are considering it. If you want an eye lift to recapture your husband's wandering gaze, I'd say your problem probably can't be solved in the OR. But if that bump on your nose has always left you with your nose out of joint, so to speak, then maybe it's worth a date with the scalpel. Whatever you are contemplating, think long and hard before you act. With age comes wisdom. (Wha'd you think I was going to say? Crow's feet?) And the focus of your anxiety today, you may not even notice tomorrow. (Or, more realistically, the day after that.)

Personally, I have spent years watching—sometimes in bemusement, other times in horror—as my face has changed. From thin to heavy (and back and forth), from young to … um, not *quite* so young. I've been so sunburned, I could have been mistaken for a long-lost Hilton sister; my skin has become so oily, I could open my own trattoria; I have rosacea and have had pimples and, Lord, everything in between. Yet I still believe that I have good skin—and I work hard to keep it that way.

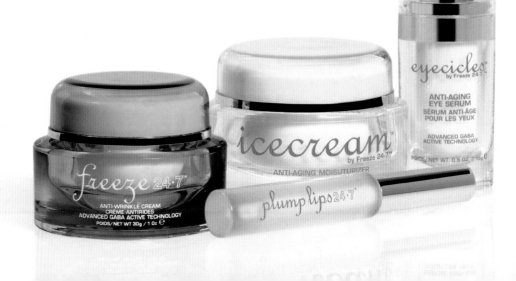

With all that said, would I go under the knife? Yep. Sure, I would. And in another few years, I just might. And if I do, you can be damn sure I'll get the best plastic surgeon I can afford, too. Let's be real: A bungled surgery will only make a bad situation worse (and potentially as painful physically as it is emotionally). But—and this is a significant "but," so pay attention—I would only sign up for a minor adjustment or two. Frankly, I like a face with a few lines on it. Wrinkles are to a person what embarrassing photos are to a party—they prove that a good time was had. In the end, isn't that what life is all about? Don't give me that malarkey about dying young and leaving a beautiful corpse, because hello?! It ain't going to be beautiful for long! One of my favorite quotes in the world is from *The Wizard of Oz*, "A heart cannot be judged by how much it loves but by how much it is loved by others." Make sure that when you reach that big checkout counter in the sky, your face registers all the laughter and tears that have made you so beloved.

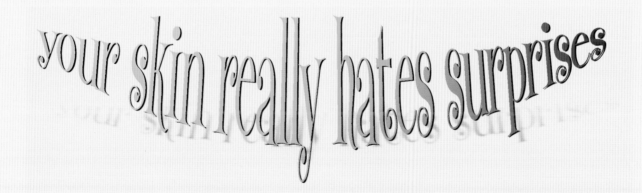

KATHY BRIER

How do I love Kathy Brier? Let me count the ways. I love her first and foremost for her talent. Sweet Jesus, when this kid sings, the angels weep (I'd say they turn on the waterworks out of envy, but I imagine cherubs are above at least most of the seven deadly sins). She also has impeccable comic timing—ask anyone who was lucky enough to catch her as the socially conscious hoofer Tracy Turnblad in Broadway's *Hairspray*. What's more, the girl is as versatile as a black mini dress! As *One Life to Live* heroine Marcie Walsh, she plays both heartbreak and hilarity with such conviction that I often want to alternately hug and hang out with her. However, the biggest reason I love Kathy has nothing to do with what she does; it's simply about who she is. You won't find her shopping in the petite section of Bloomingdale's, yet she talks the talk and walks the walk of the beautiful woman that she is. She doesn't come off like someone who goes to sleep at night sighing, "Oh, if only I could lose a few pounds …" No, she strikes me as someone who likes who she is and who knows that other people can't help but like her, too. But you can draw your own conclusions. Won't you join me in spending some time with her?

"TALENT,
DEDICATION
& PASSION
FOR YOUR
CRAFT
DON'T
ALWAYS
EQUAL
SUCCESS
OR
FAIRNESS"

KATHY BRIER

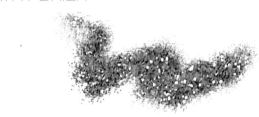

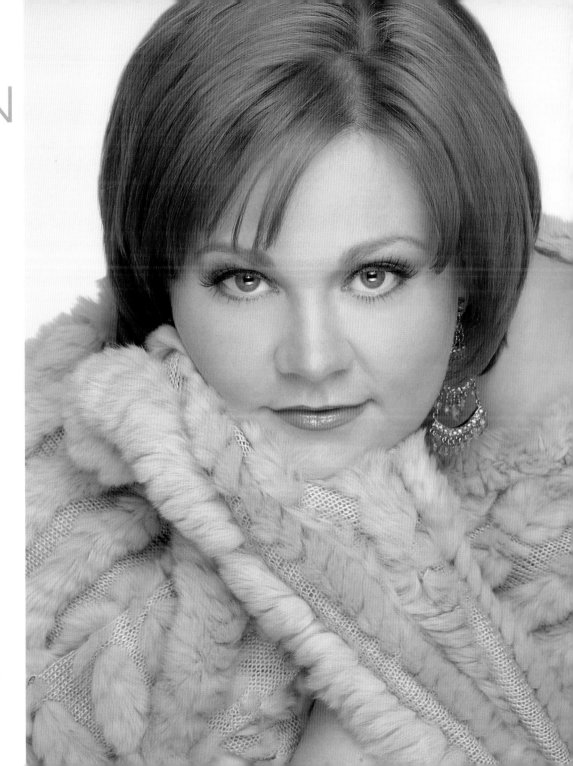

What is beauty to you?

What I find beautiful is someone who is comfortable in their own skin and also has a great sense of humor.

That right there is reason No. 204 why you are such an inspiration to me. Of course, reasons No. 205 and 206 are that you're a knockout and you're sooo cool. But I digress. What's your personal style?

My style is the things that nobody else can pull off or the things that you wouldn't expect.

Mm-hmm. There's reason No. 211. Where beauty is concerned, what do you feel like you have to hide, if anything?

I don't like my arms, but I think clothes hide a multitude of sins.

Hallelujah! Okay, come clean—do you wax, tweeze or shave?

I do a buzz! I hate waxing!

If I peeked at your appointment book—um, not that I would *ever* do something like that—what would we find listed next on your to-do list?

I'm heading to Nashville. I'm also doing a cabaret show as well as several family weddings.

Do you have any good make-up horror stories?

None yet. But I have a hair horror story.

And me without any marshmallows or a campfire! Go on.

When I was 13, I took a picture out of a magazine and went to a hair salon and showed the stylist. What I wanted was a sassy pixie cut, but when she was done, I looked like Caesar. It was horrible for the whole summer.

Hail, Kathy! What's your best make-up story?

Well, when I started at *One Life to Live*, the world of make-up was revealed to me, and at the same time, it boosted my self-confidence. It's amazing.

When you travel, what do you have to bring with you?

A pair of jeans, a cute dress—something that can be smashed into my luggage and pulled out and worn—my favorite pair of gold high heels and a bottle of water.

What is your favorite pick-me-up? And don't say love scenes with Nathaniel Marston!

Dancing, swimming and oh yeah, the beach.

What's your favorite guilty pleasure? Again, aside from love scenes with Nathaniel.

Pleasure can never be guilty, can it? No, it can't!

You've obviously never met my friends Ben and Jerry. Who are your favorite designers?

David Quinn and Tadashi.

Do you believe that make-up has power?

Yes. *One Life to Live* has taught me the power of make-up to transform you and lift your spirits as well as to enhance what's beautiful about you.

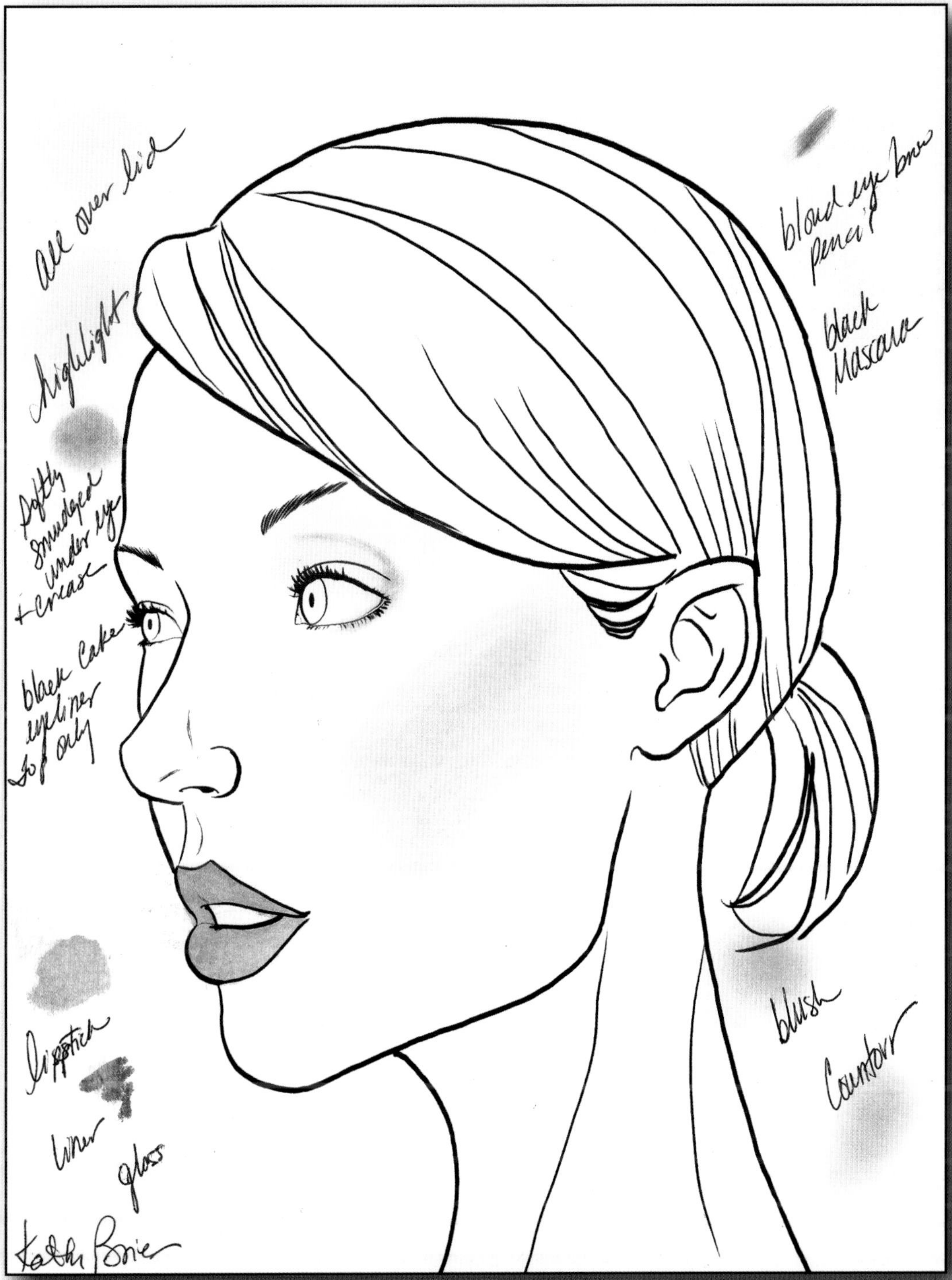

All over lid

Highlight

Softly smudged under eye + crease

black cake eyeliner top only

blond eye brow pencil

black mascara

lipstick

liner gloss

blush

contour

Who is your favorite person, dead or alive?

My grandmother. She was so ahead of her time. She was the one who taught me to follow my dreams and that all things are possible. She also gave a false age to join the Army as a nurse, and was [enlisted] at 17. She was such an inspiration.

Wow. I can imagine! On an unrelated note, what's your favorite smell?

Pumpkin … like pies. And the smell after it rains.

Favorite taste? Or do I have to ask?

Pumpkin.

At least you're consistent. Favorite sound?

The ocean.

Favorite touch?

Skin or fur.

Favorite sight?

The ocean.

What's the hardest lesson you have learned so far?

Wow. A lot of lessons, but the biggest one is that talent, dedication and passion for your craft don't always equal success or fairness for your work.

See? Your grandmother's advice is perfect—and it's truer nowadays than ever.

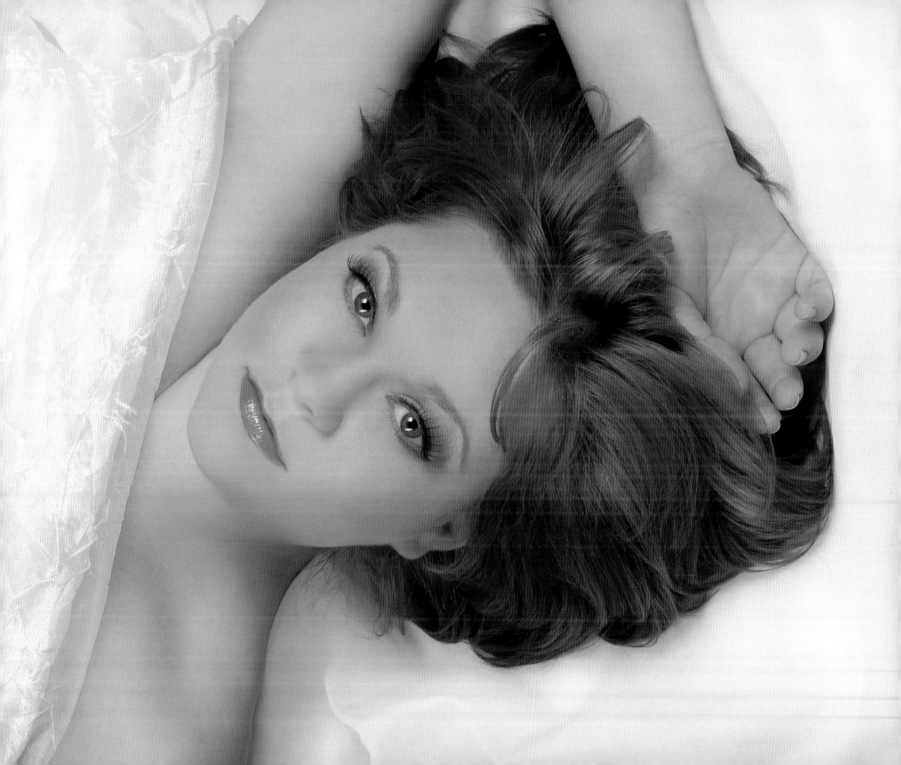

JUDI EVANS

There is something to be said for women who are mysterious and hard to read. "What is that something?" you ask. Um, mostly, they are mysterious and hard to read, which, if you ask me, is damning them with faint praise. I far prefer a gal who is an open book—better still, one with big, bold-faced print and lots of good humor. Such a fun-loving broad—and I use the term "broad" only with the greatest affection—is my pal, Judi Evans. We've been cracking up playing with make-up for more than a decade now, and unless one of us seriously ticks off the Fates, I expect we will continue doing so for at least another 10 years. No doubt, my estimation of her character will not surprise soap fans in the least. Sure, she got her start playing teary-eyed heroines (*Guiding Light*'s Beth Raines and *Days of Our Lives*' Adrienne Johnson). But it's been in her more recent roles (*Another World*'s reformed troublemaker Paulina Cory, and *Days*' social-climbing Bonnie Lockhart) that her inner wild child has been allowed—no, encouraged!—to shine through. (How much chutzpah does the Emmy winner really have? In the TV movie *Getting Away with Murder: The JonBenet Ramsey Mystery*, she tackled the part of the victim's suspicious stage mother.) Lucky for you, I'm not greedy: You're welcome to laugh along as I catch up with the extremely funny lady.

"WE NEED TO STEP BACK, TAKE A BREATH AND HAVE A LAUGH"

JUDI EVANS

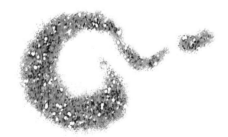

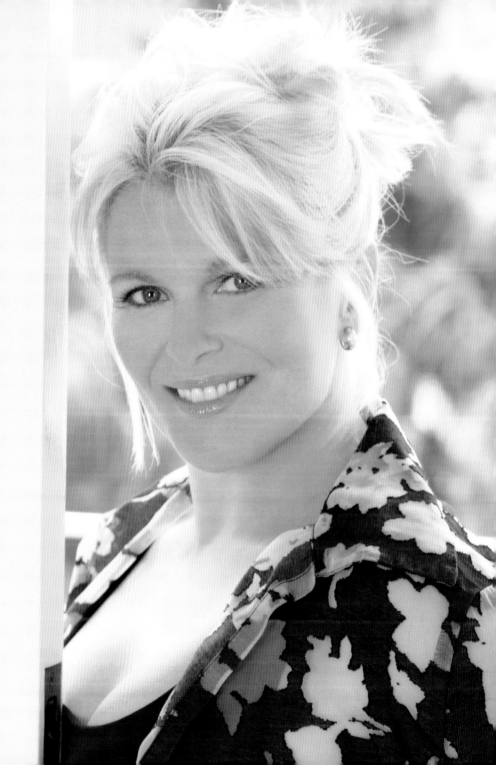

When you and I met, you were doing *Another World*, and now you're back on *Days Of Our Lives*. Is there a big difference stylewise between Paulina and Bonnie?

Oh, yes. Bonnie wears anything and everything. Paulina was edgy, but still mostly a good girl, whereas Bonnie is more mischievous. So there are lot more lashes and a lot bigger hair now!

You're a lot more Bonnie than Paulina, aren't you?

Yeah, now. *(Laughs)* I definitely am.

You're from California, and now you're living here again. Looking at you, I have to say it definitely seems to agree with you.

Thank you! I love the sunshine. I think [looking good] has to start from within. And whatever makes you feel good, you should definitely do. I'm a firm believer in that.

So, off duty, what makes you feel good? What's your personal style?

Very casual. I hardly ever wear make-up. In fact, I just put some hardening gel in my hair, to give it some oomph, and that's pretty much what I do.

Wax, tweezer or razor?

Where? *(Laughs)*

Anywhere!

Oh, wax. I love wax. I'm very hairy, so tweezing, I just go insane.

What's your favorite pick-me-up?

My family. Just being around them gets me going. Seriously.

Favorite guilty pleasure?

McDonald's French fries.

Remember when they changed them? God, that was awful!

I thought they were smart to bring them back. You need old grease, dammit! Seriously, I go to the gym just so I can have French fries at least once a week.

Besides hitting the gym, what else do you do for an audition? Do you go in au naturel or fully made up?

Depends on the character. If the character's kind of a nice girl, more natural. If the character's a little edgier, then [I'll alter my appearance]. It depends on what age I'm going in as, too. If I'm going in to play somebody younger, then a lighter make-up. But a lot of times, I go in for older roles, so I wear a little bit more.

What do you think is your best feature—and we're covering both ends of the spectrum here!

My sense of humor and my new boobs. *(Laughs)*

You want to talk about your new boobs?

I had a breast reduction and a lift, and I feel sexier than ever. I was used to being big-bosomed and I'm still big, but it took a little time for me to find this new sexiness about it, and I love it. From the neck to the upper abdomen, I'm 18.

You don't want to change anything higher than your neck—that mind of yours would be a terrible thing to waste! In your opinion, what's your worst feature?

Oh, my butt.

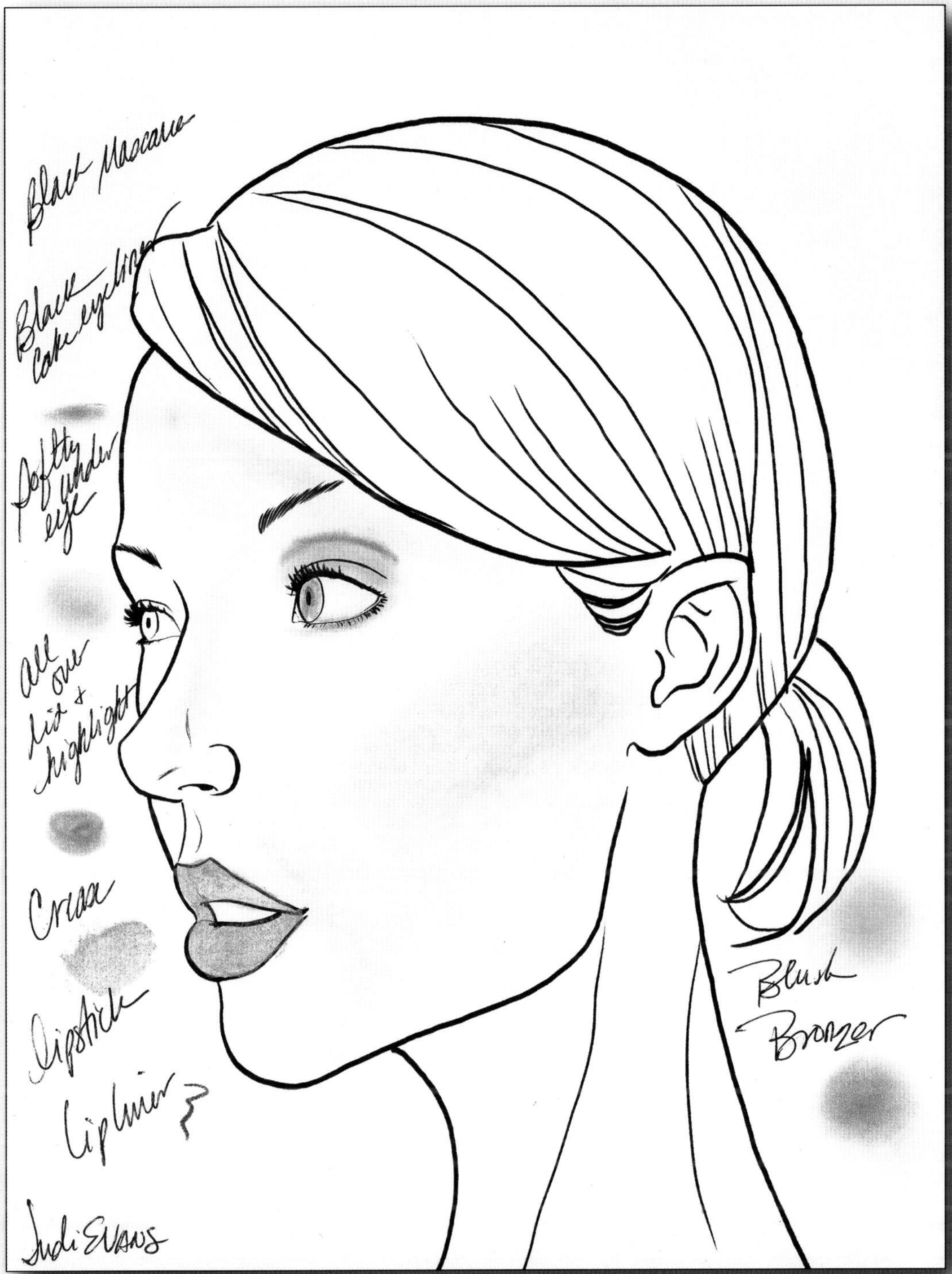

Black Mascara

Black Cake eyeliner

Softly under eye

All over lid + highlight

Crease

Lipstick

Lipliner

Blush
Bronzer

Judi Evans

Not from where I'm standing!
I don't have any booty call.

Then you're not giving your number to the right people, honey! Who taught you the most about beauty in your life?
My mother. I was born in the '60s, so I was [brought up with] lashes and liners and lipstick, big time.
Lashes, liners and lips! I was born in the circus, you know. My parents were trapeze artists.

No way!
Yes! So they always had to be glamorous.

That's too weird. I'm related to P.T. Barnum through my partner!
No way!

Way! He was a distant cousin. So we're both circus folk.
Circus *trash*.

(Laughs) When do you feel the most beautiful. Is there a particular time of day … or a point in your life?
In the morning, definitely. And …

… at night. (Snickers)
At night, in the dark. *(Laughs)* Seriously, as each decade comes along, I actually feel more beautiful and more self-assured. I'm still at an age where I can be womanly and girly at the same time, and I really like that.
Even though I'm a total tomboy, I feel girly and flirty, too.

Speaking of flirting, you sassy vixen, who's been your favorite leading man?
Oh, wow. That's a hard one. It has to be a toss-up between John Ingle (*Days* moneybags Mickey Horton)
and Joe Barbara and Tom Eplin (Paulina's husbands, Joe Carlino and Jake McKinnon, on *Another World*).
It has to be a three-way tie.

Well, if it has to be a three-way … That's the three-way to have! (Laughs) Oh my gosh!
What really gets your motor running for a guy?
Eyes, sense of humor and just raw sexuality. They have to have all three.

Gee, you don't ask for much! (Laughs) And the biggest turn-off about a guy?
Arrogance. I could smack him upside the head!

Okay, last question—what do you think is missing in the world that you once had but now miss?
A sense of innocence and fun. A sense of laughter.

Do you think that's a side effect of growing up or just a sign of the times?
It's a sign of the times. I try to interject that [into my life]—I want to make people laugh. I think some of our boundaries are too strict about making a joke about this or that. I see where [there's such a] need [for restrictions], but we've lost that '50s innocence, and we can never get that back.

We've also lost a big sense of humor. Things are so serious now. We need to step back, take a breath and have a laugh. And wear lips and lashes and liner—the three Ls!

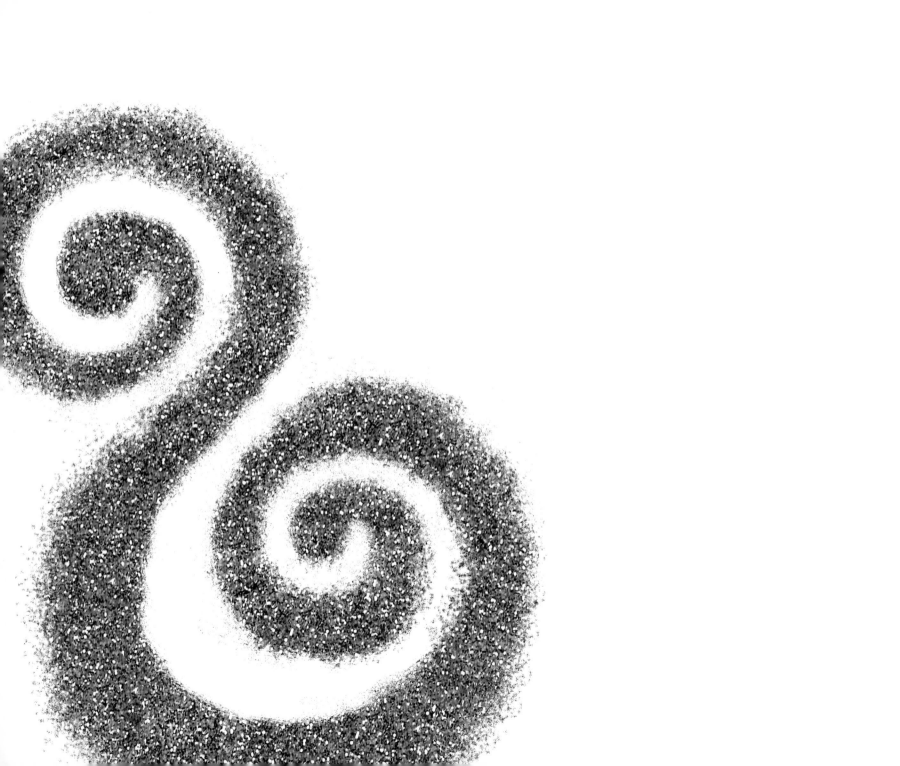

CHAPTER 3:
Put a Lid on It!

For as long as you can remember, you've heard it: The eyes are the windows to the soul. So it stands to reason that you would want to give those windows nice shutters, right? Right.

Thus, we turn our gaze to this chapter of unparalleled importance. But before we get down to the nitty-gritty (figuratively speaking, of course; one wants neither nits nor grit anywhere near one's peepers), it bears mentioning that we are not reinventing the wheel. To crib from another overused cliché, the eyes already have it; our job is merely to draw as much attention as possible to, ahem, it. I should stress here that the kind of attention we want is *positive*, not random. Yellow eyeshadow will turn heads, sure … right along with stomachs. That's why we're going to work within the color scheme of your complexion, avoiding hues that, even at its nastiest, nature never intended.

First, let's try an exercise. (No, you won't need a No. 2 pencil or even a mascara wand. Your imagination is all that's required.) Say you're having a conversation with someone, chatting away. What you're saying is important (let's hope), but *how* you are saying what you are saying is just

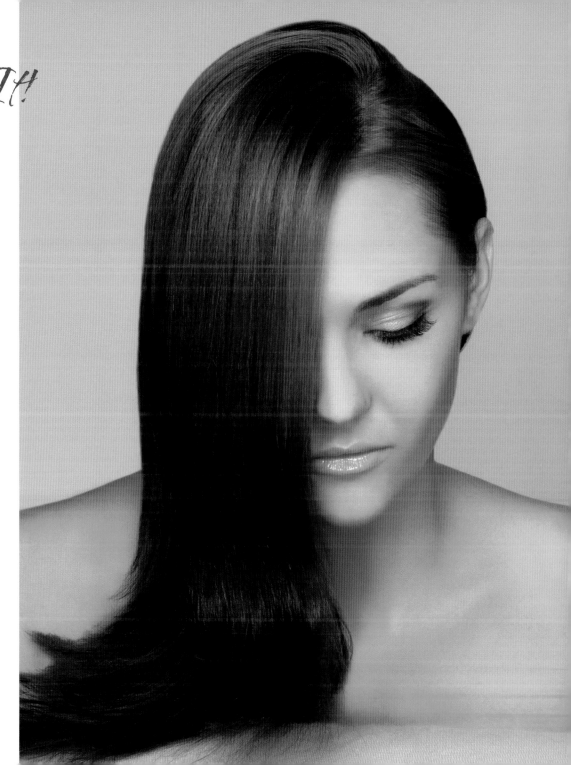

as important as *what* you are saying. (Dizzy yet?) The tone you choose, the way you gesture and, above all, the look in your eyes communicate as much, if not more, than your words. Even watching *All My Children* with the sound off, you can always tell whether Erica Kane is saying "Come 'ere, big boy!" or "Go away, little man!" simply by glancing at her eyes. The same is true of you. So, naturally, for the duration of this téte-a-téte, the last thing you want is for your companion to notice your earrings, the tablecloth or, worst of all, the cute cashier behind the counter. Don't be ashamed to admit it: You want all eyes on *you*—and the surest way to achieve that goal is by keeping all eyes on your eyes.

SHEDDING LIGHT ON EYESHADOW

Let's start with something basic, shall we? I call this look "the basic eye." (Ingenious, no?) It works all the time and is so simple to achieve that a child could pull it off, no sweat (although really, you would never want a child to apply eyeshadow—how creepy is that?). Anyway, start by looking straight into the mirror and dividing your eye into three areas: the lid, the crease and the highlight.

Our first actual step (that last bit wasn't so much a step as it was a pre-step; c'mon, work with me here, people!) is to cover the entire area with a shadow primer, a foundation-type product created to prevent creasing and camouflage veins and red or blue tones. (The primer works in much the same way as a stained-glass window— it's dark until you put light behind it, then cue the chorus of angels: Hallelujah! The eye opens right up, visually.)

Next, it's time to move into the shadows. (Nothing to be afraid of; these are femme fatale shadows, not holy-crap-it's-that-scary-guy-with-the-blue-face-from-*Passions* shadows.) Start creating your shadows with your lightest shade, then get increasingly dark. The highlight shade should cover the entire area, from your lashes to your eyebrows. Using a large fluff brush, blend as you go, and keep dusting off excess.

Next, take your crease shade and, using a medium or small fluff brush, run it across the crease while looking straight into the mirror. Go back and forth so as to slowly deepen the crease and add dimension to the area. Then, take a deeper shadow and, using a small line brush or smudger, blend the darker shade across the base of the lashes until you have achieved the desired results.

When you are done, take a cue from Stevie Nicks and stand back, stand back. Look closely at your work. Do you need to take the large fluff again and blend it all together? If so, get to it. This stuff may be as simple as coloring by numbers, but you certainly don't want the finished product to resemble a color-by-numbers masterpiece. This last little bit of "blenditure" (which is not a word but should be) will give you a soft basic eye for work or play, the classroom or the nightclub. (Naturally, for clubbing, you'll want to select a darker crease line for a more dramatic appearance. You may choose to do the same when doing especially dull research at the library— you know, just to shake things up.)

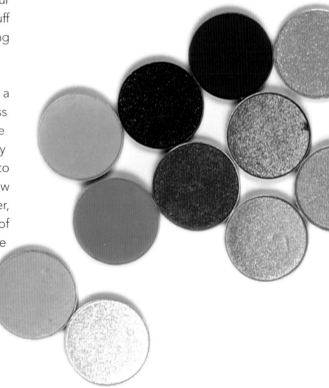

SMOKE SCREENING

Next up are smoky eyes. How sexy is that, huh? Even the name of this look evokes images of a *Casablanca* where, mysteriously, no one needs Visine to remain clear-eyed. But, just as *Casablanca* was filled with as much danger as romance, so is this look a cosmetic minefield. A step to the left, and you're gorgeous, a vamp on par with the bodacious blood-suckers of *Port Charles*; a step to the right, and you'll get mistaken for an extra from *Dawn of the Dead*. So let's proceed cautiously. *Very* cautiously.

As with basic eyes, you will need to know the three areas of the eye. They come into play again here, the only difference being the heavier shades we select. Got that? Okay. We're ready to go dark …

First, highlight the same area that you did for basic eyes. (See? This isn't so tough. You're probably already saying to yourself, "Been there, done that." It gets more exciting, though. Keep reading.) Then, use your midtone on the lid—but only on the inner half. Put the darker shade on the outer half, blending in the crease area, then slowly blend under the eye as a liner. Also, blend across the crease toward the nose. (Told you it got trickier.) If you suddenly look about as hot as a cadaver, take a blush shade and run it across the top of the crease, and blend like your life depended on it. Adding this extra shadow goes a long way toward softening this harsher look. (So do eyeliner and mascara. Quit stomping your Manolos; we'll get there.)

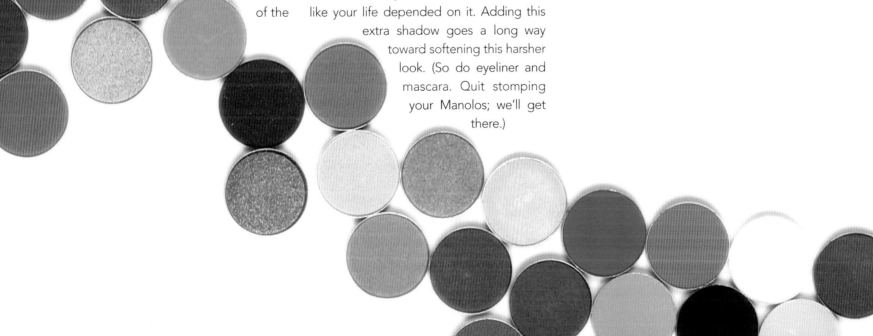

WHAT'S MY LINE?

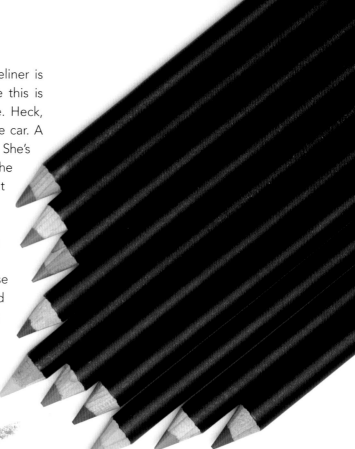

See? I told you we'd get to eyeliner. Now, the thing to remember about eyeliner is that it is supposed to make your lashes look fuller while subtly reshaping or outlining the contour of the eye.

Go back and read that last line again. No whining, just do it, please, because it is important. Anything you try to get out of your eyeliner over and above those two results, you must acknowledge, at least to yourself, is just for fun. Got it? You can try it. You can mess around with it. But when you end up looking like you've been painted up for a very special Halloween episode of *One Life to Live*,

don't come cryin' to me. (I mean, for starters, that eyeliner will run all over the place.)

Now that we've got *that* out of the way, I'll confess that I like a cake eyeliner with a little brush—yes, the one that everybody insists they can't possibly use. This just in: You *can* use it, but like everything else, it takes practice. Take, for example, my sister. She's an au naturel sort—pretty as a peach, but about as skillful with make-up as I am with a chainsaw.

Yet even she thinks that cake eyeliner is a piece of … oh, you see where this is going. Insert your own joke here. Heck, you should see her apply it in the car. A couple of seconds, and va-voom! She's good to go until she removes the stuff. (It's nice and semi permanent that way.)

I especially like to use cake eyeliner when going for the smoky-eye look. You can even use your little brush to subtly blend eyeshadow into the liner, cutting the edge off a little—because subtlety is the name of the game.

LASHING OUT

You know how important it is that your hair have just the right curl? (Unless you are Cher, circa 1976.) Well, it's just as important that your eyelashes have the right curl. (Don't worry; it's not like plucking nose hairs—it's painless and fun. And for once, even though it's coming from a man, you can believe that line.)

Now then, when "lashing out," as it were, the first step is to use a lash curler to softly bend your lashes up toward your eyebrows. Start close to the lash base (by the lid), then slowly move the curler out in one-quarter-inch increments until your lashes are as upturned as your smile (or as upturned as you like—some people have *really* big smiles). While you're at it, don't forget the inner and outer corner lashes. For one thing, they sulk when they are neglected. For another, they will punish you for your neglect

by making you look one-tenth less stunning. (Or something like that—eyelashes have never been very good at percentages.)

Once you're done there, it's time to apply your mascara. Should you go with waterproof or not? That all depends. If you are a soap actress whose character is prone to crying fits, then yes, by all means, get waterproof. Otherwise, you may not need it. All kidding aside, the deciding factor is how you plan to remove the mascara: If you are using an eye make-up remover, then waterproof is preferable; if you intend to shower it off, choose the regular kind. (Just a reminder—yes, I know, I'm a terrible nag—you should always remove your make-up at bedtime. Among other benefits, your lashes will be healthier and, thereby, in better condition for batting.)

Now before we begin, a quick quiz: What is an eyelash? (No, that is not a *Jeopardy!* style answer but the question at hand.) Although "something you wish on" and "that thing that always gets wedged between my eye and my contact lens" are both fine answers, the one I was looking for was … a hair. Yep, much like the kind on your head. As such, lashes are round. Knowing this will help you to realize that

your lashes have sides as well as tops and bottoms.

When applying mascara, start at the top of the hair. Slide the mascara wand down over the top of the lashes, then come up the bottom. If you would like a thicker coat, go on to place the wand at the base of the hair and wiggle it back and forth for a few seconds, so as to place a little extra product there. (Try it, you'll like it—this technique produces really glorious results.) Next, take a lash comb and slide it through to the ends of the lashes, along the way removing any clumps and separating the hairs so that the lashes look as individual as the woman wearing them. (Quick trick: For maximum magic production, wipe your wand on a tissue before starting; this will remove the excess mascara that would normally clump.)

Once you are satisfied with your work, sit back and let those lashes flutter as you feign surprise at all the hoopla your eye-catching orbs have provoked.

EYE CARAMBA!

Before we move on, I would like to offer you one last little tip. Whether you go for basic or smoky eyes, or something in between, what people should notice is your eye color, not your make-up. Those limpid pools ought to appear vibrant and alive, sparkling and mischievous (unless you have something against mischief, in which case they should appear sparkling and, um, modest?). Your make-up design should only enhance, never overpower, your eyes.

Allow me to illustrate. I'd ask you to close your eyes and concentrate, but that would make reading a bit difficult. Instead, simply picture your living room. If it is blue, and you add a blue chair or a blue rug or a blue lamp, they will be just that: blue. However, if you buy a gold chair and/or rug and/or lamp, you will have done a brilliant job of contrasting—creating interest by encouraging the different hues to make you say, "Viva la difference!" The blue will seem bluer and the gold, more golden. Cool, huh? And you can do the same thing with your eyes. Stop, look and look again: See which shades pump up *your* volume, then let 'er rip!

By the way, you can also see excellent examples of contrast in any ad for the "latest, greatest eye make-up" of the month: The colors being marketed are almost always soft, but the hues used in the backdrops? Saturated with bold shades. I've been fooled more times than I choose to admit by that kind of ad—and those of you who have drawers full of misfit cosmetics know the pain of which I speak. Everything always looks different at home, and this is why!

In closing, I would like to add that, as much as we may enhance the look of your eyes with make-up, what is, always has been and always shall be important about them is what is behind them: your heart and soul, your wisdom and strength. I learned so much more from the women in my (actual and extended) family than the importance of eyebrow shaping and lip liner, and I'd wager my favorite fluff brush that they would agree that no lesson was more critical than the one about the gilding being all but insignificant to the lily's beauty. That's why it breaks my heart when I see women who let their nearest and dearest (who are also some times their meanest and nastiest) run them down and cripple their self esteem. There is nothing so lovely, or as profound, as a woman who has found her core … who has found herself and realized that what is special about her doesn't come in a tube or compact. (And, while we're on the subject, it doesn't fluctuate with diet and exercise, either.) It's inside of you, so accept that and remember it, and you should come through your experiments with yellow eyeshadow—and all of life's trials—with flying colors.

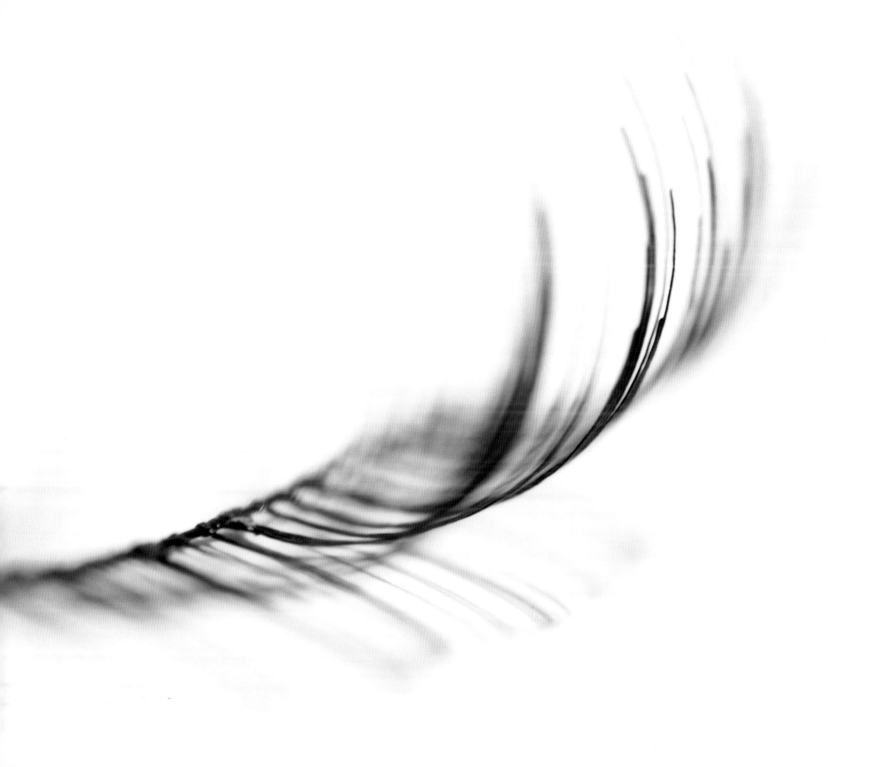

ILENE KRISTEN

When I met Ilene Kristen, I could tell right away that she was old school: The woman knows how to make an entrance! She breezed into her photo session and proceeded to pull out of her bag one peasant dress after another after another. (If she'd had one more garment stuffed into that thing, I swear to God I was going to ask her do all my packing forevermore!) But her larger-than-life persona would come as no surprise to anyone who's ever seen her work. Although she's most fondly remembered as *Ryan's Hope* troublemaker Delia—she also left an impression on viewers of *Loving* (as Norma Gilpin), *Another World* (as Madeline Thompson) and *One Life to Live*. (She's played two parts on *OLTL*: Back in the 80s, she replaced her old *Ryan's Hope* co-star, *Deep Space Nine* alien Nana Visitor, as Georgina Whitman; nearly two decades later, she returned to the show to steal scenes as underdog booze-hound Roxy Balsom.) In addition, the natural born multi-tasker has appeared on Broadway (originating the role of busybody Patty Simcox in *Grease*), in primetime shows (among them *The Sopranos*) and in films (like the indie film *Tinsel Town*). And, of course, somewhere along the way, she apparently learned how to bend the confines of space to suit her needs. Care to listen in on our conversation? Read on …

"IF IT'S NOT PRETTY ON THE INSIDE, NOBODY'S GOING TO CARE ABOUT THE OUTSIDE FOR LONG"

ILENE KRISTEN

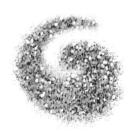

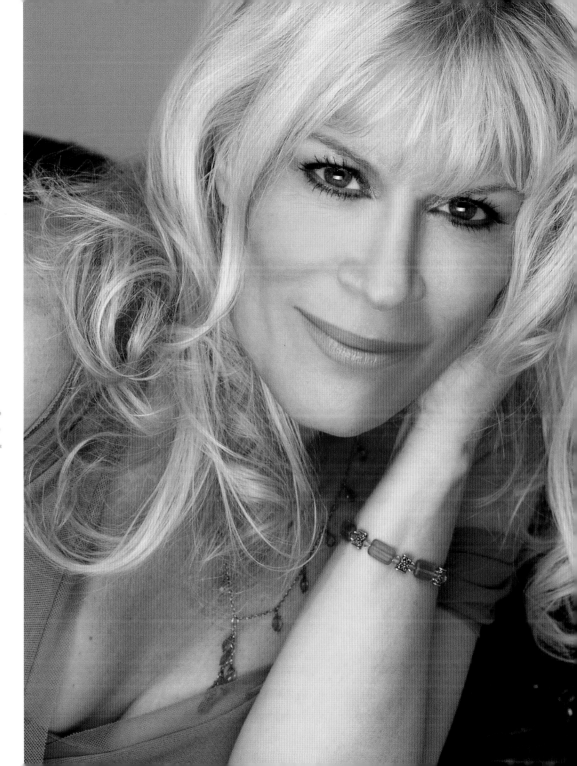

What does beauty mean to you?

It means shining your inner light out … and when you resonate beauty.

Tell me about your personal style.

My style is something I call bohemian eclectic.

Funny—I've decorated my house in a style I call bohemian hectic! What is your beauty secret?

Chinese herbs from a company called Sun Rider.

If we peeked into your appointment book, what would it say is next on your to-do list?

Pay my bills. Really! Pay my bills.

Ah, the glamorous life of a soap star! Tell me your best make-up story.

Well, I did it myself. I played the mother of an Eastern Indian girl once.
I had a black wig and a dark base. It was so bizarre. I loved it.

I've always said no make-up artist can ever know an actress' face as well as the actress herself. When you travel, what are your staples?

Oh my! Too many. Depends if I am having a curly-hair or straight-hair day … if I'm in or out …
Let's just say I don't pack lightly and leave it at that.

Consider it left. Do you believe make-up has power?

The *right* make-up has power. I have been around make-up most of my life;
my father was a hair stylist and my mother was a wardrobe stylist.

Lucky you—my household was made up of a military man and a bunch of electrical contractors! When do you feel the most beautiful?

Always during photo shoots

What is the make-up product you hate using the most?

Powder. I can't stand it. I just wish they could invent a power that would not cake or crease.
They are either too this or too that.

Funny—I often say the same thing about my relatives! What is the hardest lesson you have learned so far?

That you must save your money.

Especially around bill-paying time. Do you like false eyelashes?

Not normally; mostly during photo shoots. But I did wear them all through high school.

What are you most proud of?

My survival instincts.

If you survived high school in false eyelashes, *obviously* your survival instincts are spot-on! What storyline did you have the most fun doing?

On *One Life to Live*, Roxy's surprise marriage to Max. We filmed it for live TV.
It was amazing to do it with a live audience.

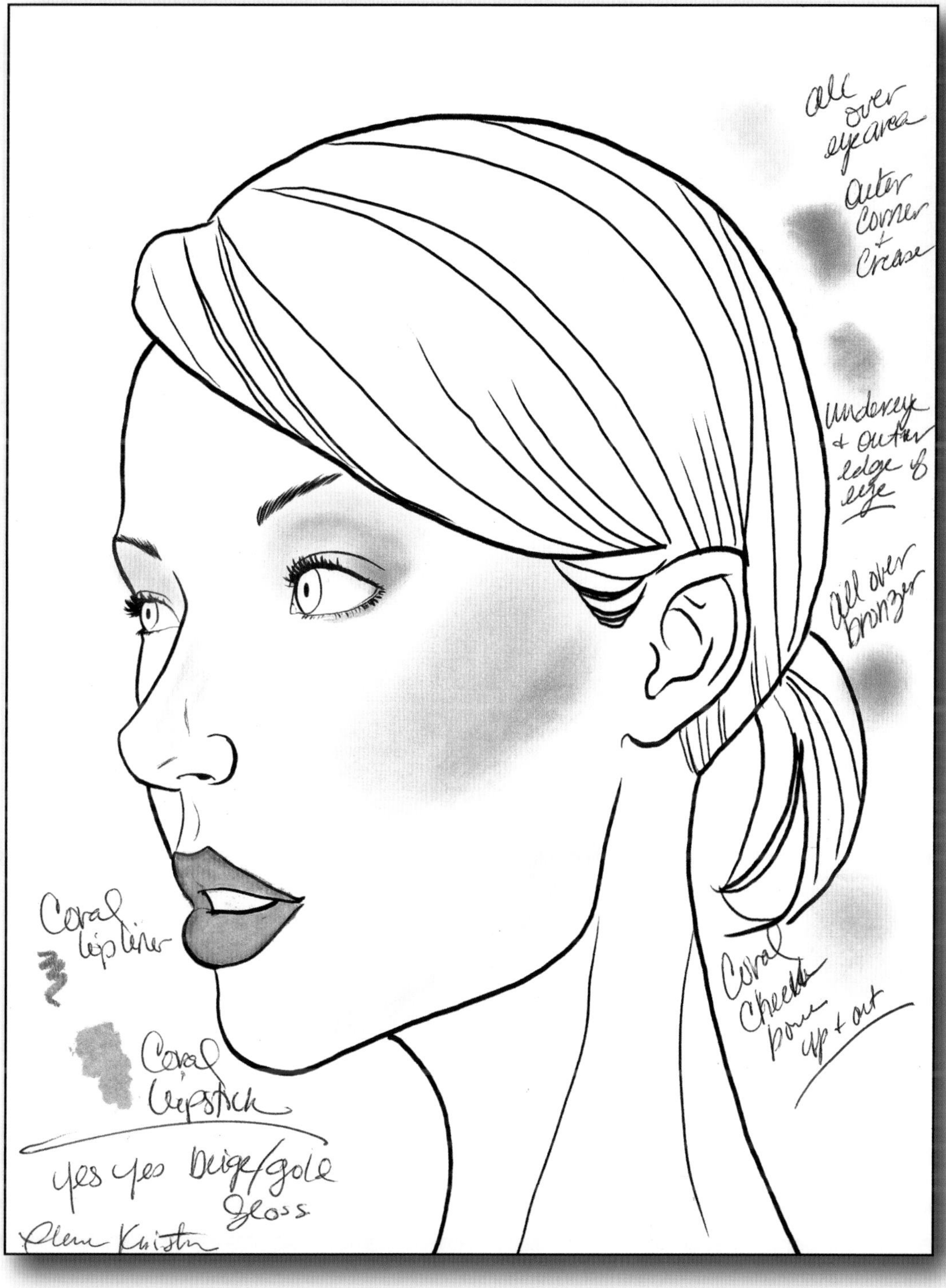

all over
eye area

Outer
Corner
+
Crease

undereye
+ outer
edge of
eye

All over
bronzer

Coral
lip liner

Coral
lipstick

yes yes beige/gold
gloss

Dear Kristin

Coral
Cheeks
bone
up + out

What is the most beneficial thing that working in daytime has afforded you?

Investments … my apartment.

Who is your favorite male co-star?

Jim DePaiva (formerly *OLTL*'s Max) and Ron Hale (who played Delia's on-again/off-again lover, Roger, on *Ryan's Hope* and now appears on *General Hospital* as Sonny and Courtney's dad, Mike).

Do you read beauty books?

Yes. Anything on anti-aging and Chinese herbs.

Do you have any hidden talents that fans might not know about?

Social work. I have in the past worked with a homeless shelter and homeless children.

That may be more of a gift than a talent—to yourself as well as to those you help out. Still, it certainly bears mentioning. Who is the person you most look to for advice or strength?

Three or four elderly women, in their 70s. And my mother.

What's missing in the world today that you once had and now miss?

A 70s sense of the world, liberal places and being free from worry.

What do you think is the most important thing for young women today to know about the myth of beauty?

That beauty comes from the inside. If it is not pretty on the inside, nobody's going to care about the outside for long.

Paris Hilton, are you paying attention? No, that's nasty. Bad me! What is your secret weapon to win over the male species?

Compassion.

What is the best gift you have ever been given?

[The ability] to accept change without kicking and screaming, and to learn from it.

You've got that one licked? Maybe you can teach me sometime. I know it's on my to-do list … somewhere.

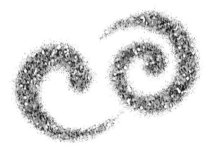

CRYSTAL HUNT

Ya either got it or ya ain't, and trust me, folks—Crystal Hunt has got it. Apparently, she always has, too. She's been working the pageant circuit since she was six months old, and before she could even get a learner's permit, she had done features like *Problem Child II* and *Homeless Children* (which I assume is not a cautionary tale about what happens to kids like the one in the former's title). Heck, she even won the gig most coveted by every starlet under the age of 30: She filmed an anti-drug PSA with 'N Sync! But in my humble opinion, we are just beginning to really appreciate the gifts with which this cobalt-blue-eyed babe has been blessed. A relative newcomer to *Guiding Light* as snobbish and some-time psycho Lizzie Spaulding, she never fails to leave me flummoxed. (Do I want to throttle the brat … or hug her? From moment to moment, I just can't decide, Crystal is so good at walking the fine line between love and hate.) In real life, Crystal just plain makes me dizzy. An apple-cheeked jumping bean, she moves a mile a minute and talks at that same pace! Luckily, you can read highlights from our conversation as slowly as you like.

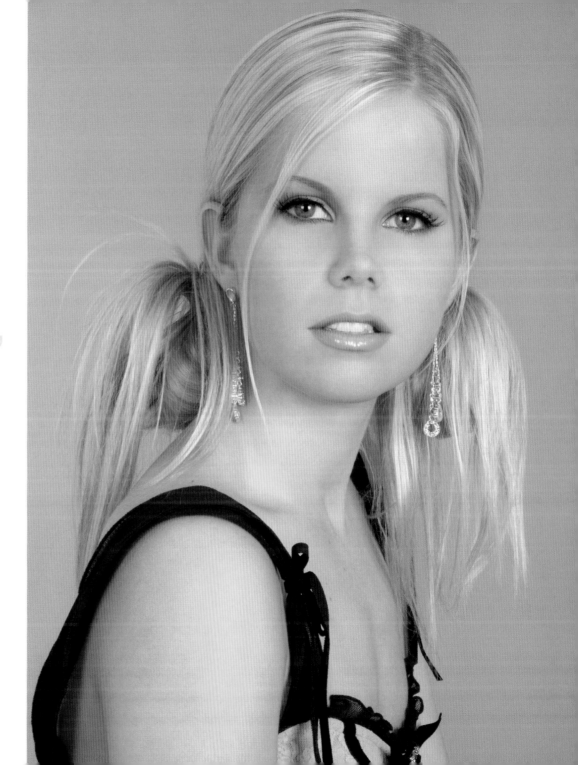

"IF YOU WANT SOMETHING, DON'T SETTLE; GO AND GET IT"

CRYSTAL HUNT

What does beauty mean to you?

You never know when the fans will be around—they want glamour, and I deliver all the time! *(Laughs)*

My hero! What's your personal style?

My style is a lot of things—basically whatever I like, especially if it's pink.

What is your secret beauty product—you know, the one you can't live without?

Lip gloss and bronzer.

Spoken like a true 19-year-old! Do you have a real-life make-up horror story?

Yes. I stopped at the counter of a store which will remain nameless, and the girl started putting make-up on me. I could tell it was awful, so I told her that I forgot I had an appointment. I bought some things and quickly left.

Never underestimate the importance of a good escape route. On the flip side, what's you best make-up story?

All the time! I just love make-up.

I believe it. You brought more cases of make-up to this photo shoot than I *own*. What's your favorite pick-me-up?

Starbucks.

I've only been with you for what? Two days? And already, I can see that you're hooked. We must've run out for coffee 50 times! But I digress. What's your favorite feature?

My blue eyes and small nose.

And your least favorite?

Oily skin.

Who is your favorite person, dead or alive?

Lucille Ball.

What's the hardest lesson you have learned so far in your life?

That you can't trust everyone.

What are you most proud of?

My family.

What do you think *Guiding Light* fans need to know about you that they don't already know?

That I'm actually a very nice and energetic person.

I can attest to that. Speaking of nice people, who do you most look to for strength and advice?

My mother, as well as Marj Dusay (who plays Lizzie's great-aunt, Alexandra) and Ron Raines (who plays her grandfather, Alan).

Your philosophy of life?

If you want something, don't settle; go and get it.

Obviously, you've taken that philosophy to heart! Which begs another question. I've met your mom, and I love her energy—I can see where you get yours! But how did she keep you in line as a kid?

She would say whenever I was bad that we were going to leave the business, and I would start crying, "No, no … !" Then she'd let me continue. I've always wanted to do acting, modeling and pageants.

Well, you must've been a beautiful baby, because baby, take a look at you now!

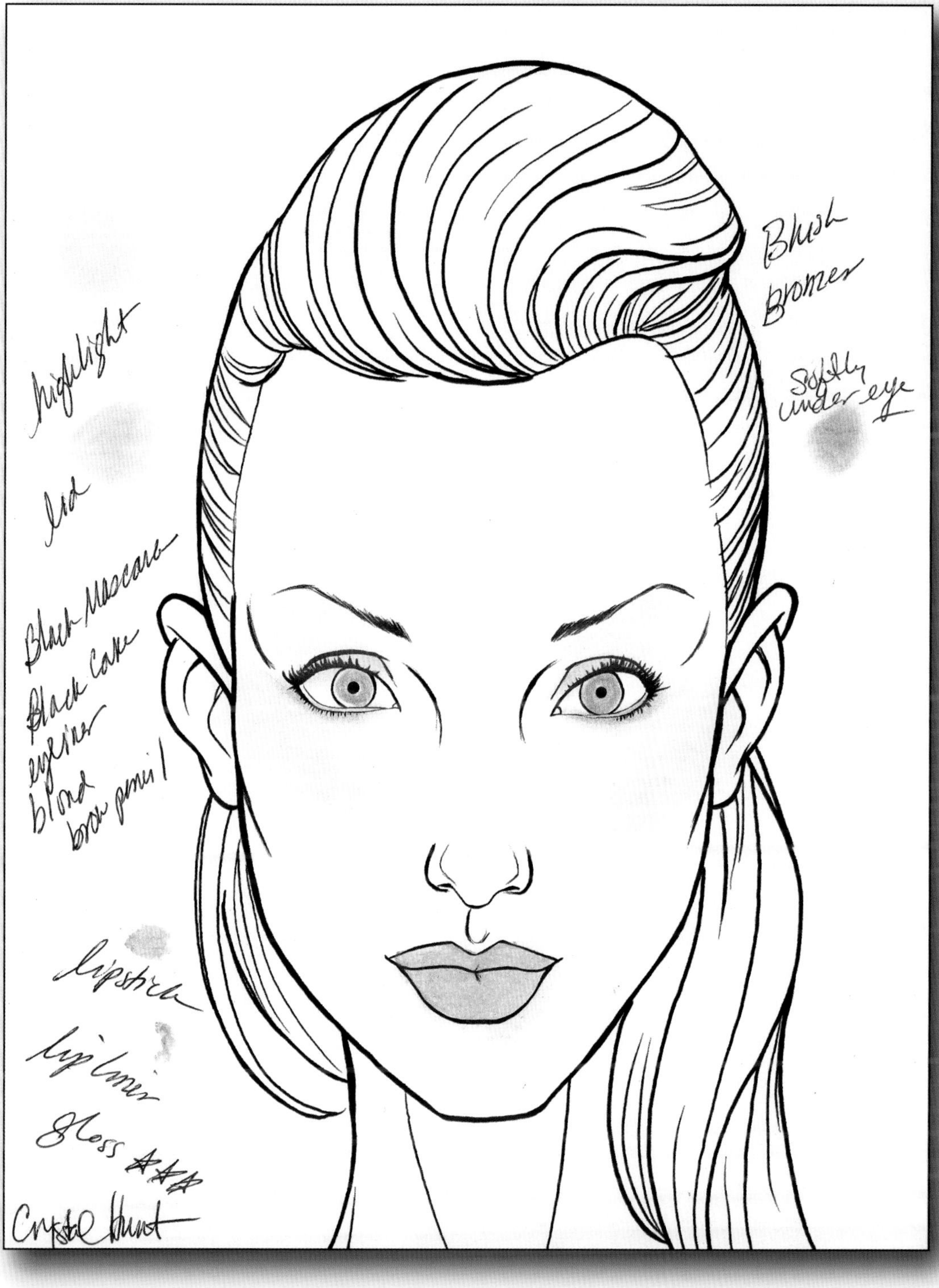

Blush
Bronzer

Softly
under eye

highlight

lid

Black Mascara
Black Cake
eyeliner
blond
brow pencil

lipstick

lip liner

gloss ###

Crystal Hunt

CHAPTER 4:

Just Browsing

Had Shakespeare been a modern woman instead of a Renaissance man, the question would not have been "To be or not to be?" but "To wax or to tweeze?"

And I would have been able to answer it for him … er, her: both. I like (and by "like," I mean "prefer," because c'mon, nobody *likes* getting a wax job!) waxing first to remove the bulk of the hair, then, if any dare to remain, a good pluck. Note: Pluck only after combing out the hair to make sure that enough is left to be arranged in the shape you require; nothing is quite as tragic as the eyebrow combovers that result from premature pruning.

How do you decide how much of a trim you need? Try this. When you have a few spare moments one day—really look at your brows. Are they too heavy? Too thin? An unruly mess? Or do they just need a trim and a little filler? While pondering these mysteries of life, use a brow brush or a clean toothbrush to give your brows a good once-over, brushing them up and out. Do you like what you see? If so, just clean them up by trimming excessively long hairs with hair or nail scissors, and accept that other women will debate whether your brows are au naturel

forevermore. If you *don't* like what you see, get thee to a pro, as the Bard would say, and get your brows waxed. If for any reason you can't avail yourself of a pro's services, then read on carefully! I'll talk you through a truly daunting salvage mission. Brace yourself. The results will be pretty, but everything that comes before you get there? Well … Not so much.

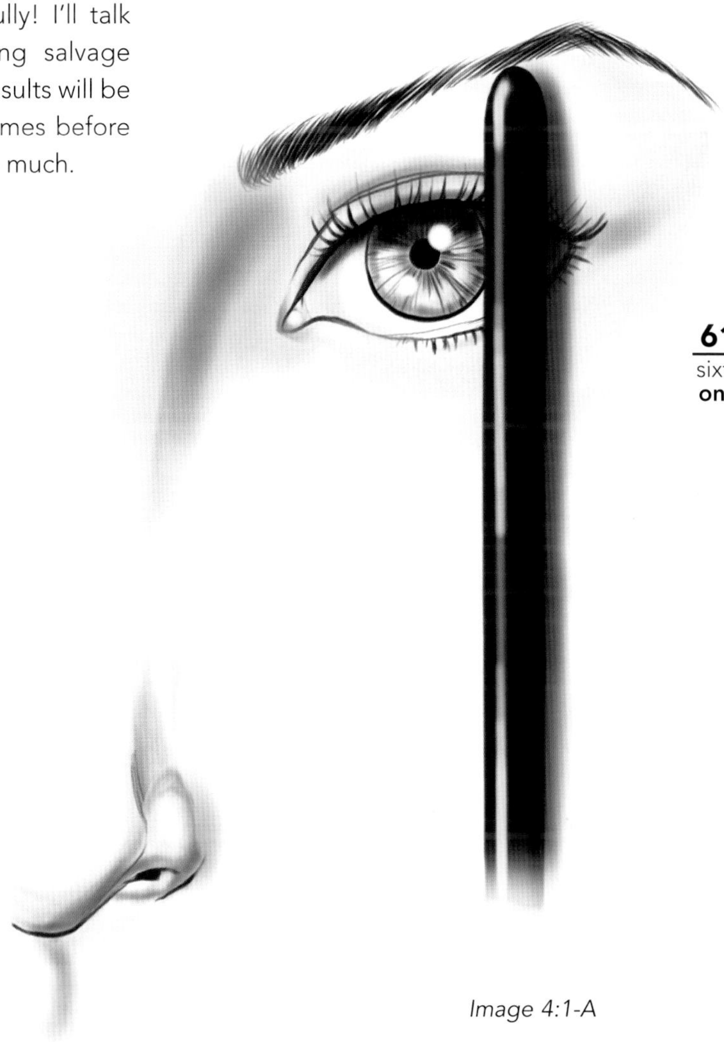

Image 4:1-A

Start by looking straight into the mirror, at the outer side of your iris (*Image 4:1-A*). This is the area above which your arch should bend (or, more simply put, the highest part of the brow). Place the handle of a make-up brush there. (A pencil will also work. A *make-up* pencil. C'mon, work with me here!) Hang in there; there are only two more steps. Place the same brush (or pencil) alongside your nose, heading up (*Image 4:1-B*). That is where your brow should begin. (And you thought you'd never use geometry in real life! Ha.) Last, to see where the brow should end, just take the pencil and make an angle from the nose to the outer corner of the eye (*Image 4:1-C*), and voila! You'll see that the pencil is going past the eye—right to the area where the brow should stop. Keep in mind that, in order to be most flattering to the face, the brow should be tapered at the end.

Okay, breathe. It wasn't *that* tough, was it? I hope nobody put out an eye, because first of all, ow, and secondly, that would make it a lot harder to appreciate your soon-to-be-achieved magnificence. Anyway, once you have a brow shape that you like, maintain it, and you'll never have to go through this kind of mind-screw torture again. And remember—what was true for the tortoise is also true of hot chicks: They go slow (in the case of hot chicks, I mean when plucking). You can always pluck more, but unplucking? Not

so easy (as all of you who have ever had to wait for badly plucked brows to grow back in can attest). And if the shape is good but you want a more powerful, or sharper, look, simply add some filler with a pencil or a shadow. (Not *too* dark, though, okay? The Joan Crawford look went out with … well, Joan Crawford.) You'll need a stiff brush for this kind of filling, because some strength is required to create particular shapes, especially like the ones you see in these images.

Image 4:1-B

Last but not least, what if the pain is second only to childbirth? (A lie, by the way: From what I hear, a bikini wax comes in second.) If you are tender and this process hurts a lot, or if you start tearing up, use ice to numb the area, and make certain that you are using a good tweezer. (You wouldn't perform surgery with a dull butter knife, would you? Then don't perform this kind of delicate operation with the wrong tool, either!) I like the slant-tip tweezer and always pull the hair in the direction in which it is already growing. (In other words, if the hair is pointing toward your hairline, pull it in that direction.) That way, the hair will come out with less discomfort. Mind you, you may still have to live up to the saying, "You have to suffer to be beautiful." But maybe by applying these pain-killing techniques, you at least won't have to suffer *quite* so much.

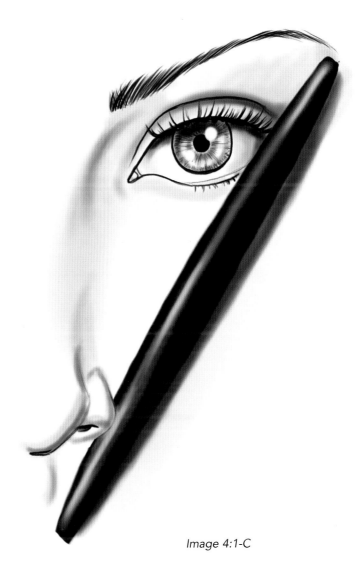

Image 4:1-C

SILVANA ARIAS

If I never learn any other words in Spanish, I now have committed to memory the two I will always like best: Silvana Arias. Prior to joining *Passions* last year as spitfire Paloma Lopez-Fitzgerald, the Peruvian-born actress was a junior achiever in telenovelas. *Maria Emilia. Gata Salvaje. Pobre Diabla. Soledad. Amor Descarado.* She's done 'em all. Yet this daughter of a respected theater actor isn't one of those know-it-all showbiz brats that you'd sooner smack than applaud. She's adorable—literally a bundle of joy. And while she insists that she struggles with English, she speaks the language beautifully (and her phrasing only makes whatever she is saying that much more enchanting). Frankly, I can't imagine anyone walking away from an encounter with her without some kind of contact high. (Casting directors, consider yourselves forewarned!) In fact, just reading through this transcript of my chat with her, I bet you'll get a nice buzz. Try it and find out.

"BEAUTY IS HOW YOU FEEL, HOW YOUR SOUL IS"

SILVANA ARIAS

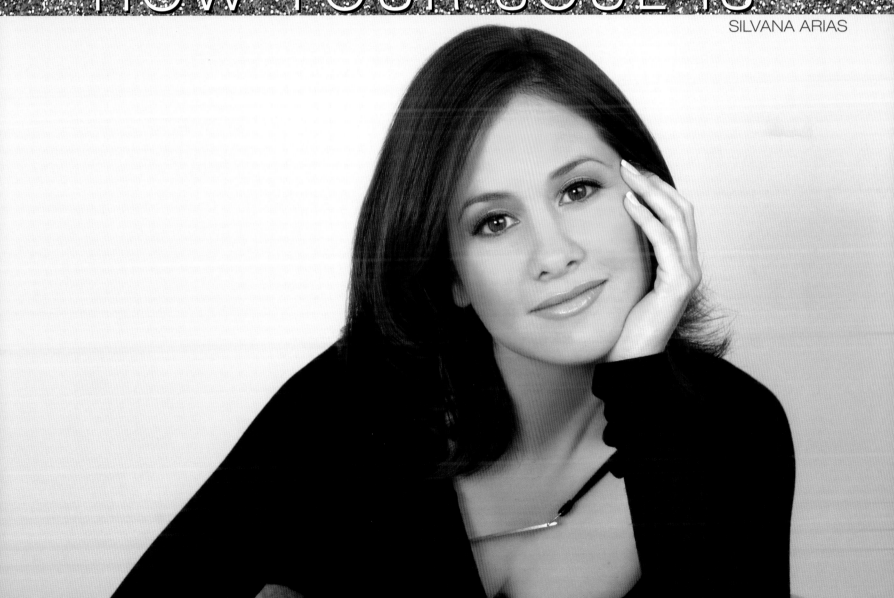

Even though I rarely understand what's going on, I love watching telenovelas. From your unique perspective, how are they different from English-language soaps?

Well, the basic difference is the telenovela has an end. The soap operas in English keep on going and going. People watching Spanish shows see the actors playing different roles in different telenovelas, and here in America, they see the same actor doing the same role for years. So people can grow up with the actors—they're like family.

Sure. Look at Susan Lucci. I think *All My Children*'s Erica was her first role, and now she's been at it for 30 years.

Oh, that's a lot. So the people think that character is part of their life. But Spanish telenovelas are fun, too, because we work a lot on location. If we have a scene in the jungle, we have to go to the jungle to do the scene, so you get more in the character.

Do you miss doing shows all in Spanish?

Sometimes, but I'm having a lot of fun with *Passions*. I like challenges, and this is my first job in English.

Really? How long have you been in the States?

Two years. And it's been only seven months since I came to Los Angeles.

Wow. Your English is really excellent!

Oh, ask [*Passions*' publicist]—my English was really, really bad when I first got here. I studied English from when I was 6 until I was 11, then I never spoke English again. Then I studied Portuguese, so I forgot a little English. But now I practice it a lot. I'm getting better, I hope. *(Laughs)*

Get any better, and you'll be better than me! I know your character has calmed down a little since she started on the show. Would you like to see her get back to being the wild child?

Yes, yes. She's just growing up. *(Affects an old-lady voice)* She's not an old lady. *(Laughs)* So I want to see her with friends and living the good life. I want her to be ... I don't know if symbol is the right word ... of the girls that come to this country and have the freedom and the opportunities that we don't have in Latin America.

A role model?

A role model, yes. I want her to show the people here that we have this freedom and this great future if you take advantage of the opportunities here. So I want Paloma to study to be better, to love her family.

So it's not just acting for you—you want to send a message.

Yes, yes, I think that actors with our characters, we should give a message to the people who are watching us, because even though [a character is] bad, [they are] not bad just because [they're] bad; they have a reason to be bad. They have a past. So, if I kill someone in the show, I don't want people to say, "Oh, okay, she killed someone, so I can kill someone." I want the message that I would be sorry for what I did.

You are now the official embodiment of this book.

What's embodiment?

You are basically merging your two worlds, the telenovelas and the soaps here. When I started using the phrase "two-faced" in writing the treatment for this book, I wanted to introduce the characters and the real women behind them to the fans. So I'm really excited that you're doing this. You're it! Now let's talk about you a bit. What does beauty mean to you?

It's the way you feel inside. It's not how you look, because we change every day. You can't stop the clock. *(Laughs)* So beauty is how you feel, how your soul is. If you're at peace, I think you look pretty.

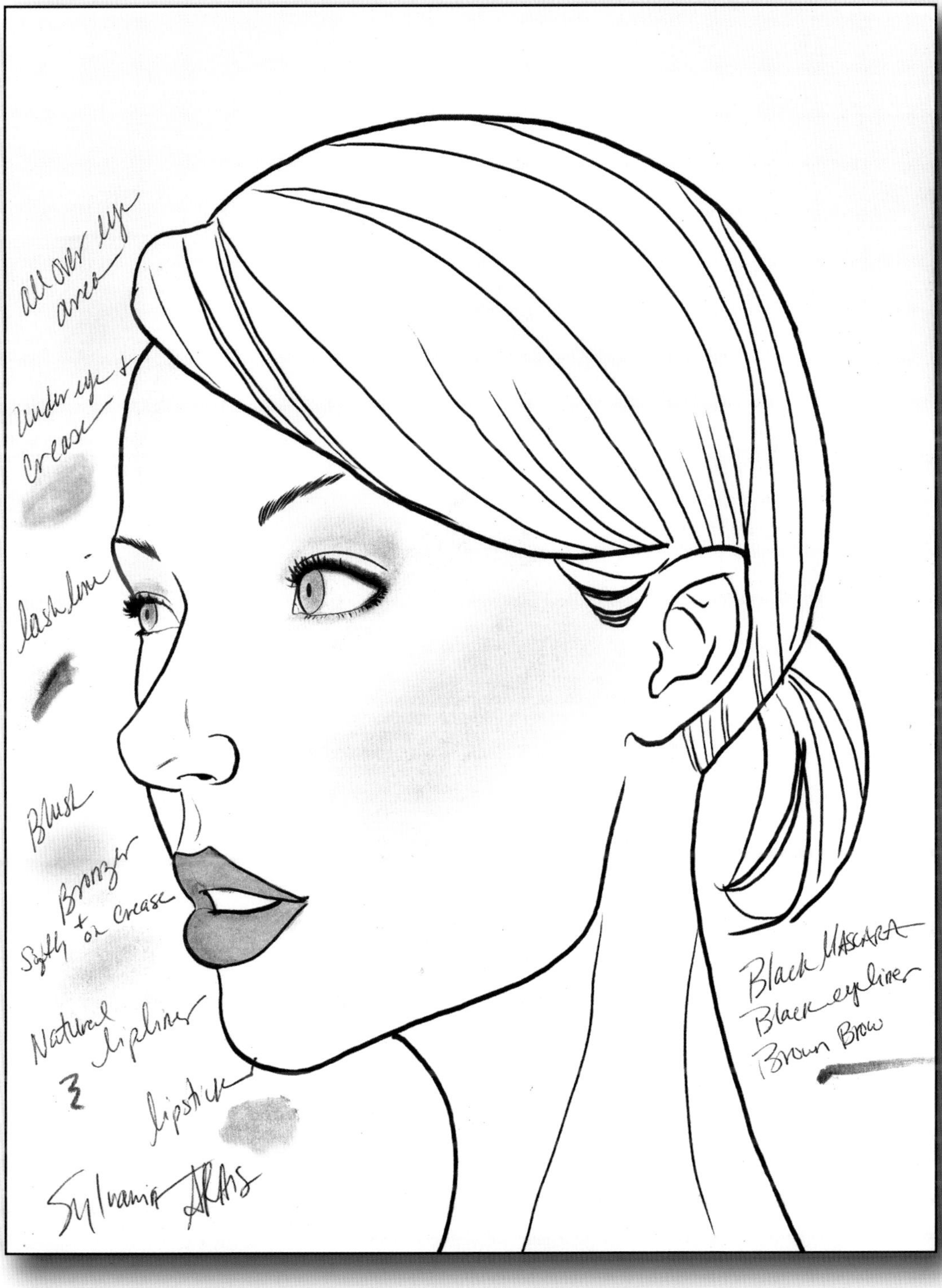

all over eye
area

under eye +
crease

lash line

Blush

Bronzer
Softly on crease

Natural lipliner
3

lipstick

Black MASCARA
Black eyeliner
Brown Brow

Sylvania ARAIS

When do you feel the most beautiful?

When I'm with my family. When I smell a good perfume. When I laugh.

You seem to do that a lot.

Yes. *(Laughs)* I'm always pretty. I'm always laughing. Sometimes there are smells that make me feel pretty, too—the fresh bread that comes from the oven … it reminds me of my country when we used to go in the morning and buy the bread with my grandmother. That makes me feel pretty.

What's your favorite make-up product?

I'm trying a face mist. It's really good.

Are you a no-make-up girl, a little-make-up girl or a lotta-make-up girl?

A little. I use make-up from Monday to Friday, so when I have to use make-up, I just like a little unless it's for pictures.

We talked a little before about your desire to be a role model. What do you think is a message for young girls who are just starting to wear make-up?

I think they have to protect their skin from the sun. I see a lot of people not using protection, and I think they need to. Also, drink a lot of water. I think you should try to take care of your skin, because you can see with a lot of products that are not good that you begin to break out. You can wear any make-up, but if your skin is not good, it's not going to look good. And your skin is the biggest organ of the body, so you have to take care of it!

At what age did you realize the power of being a woman? Or maybe it hasn't happened yet.

Well, I can't wait to turn 40, because I think …

I think you've got a lot of years to go!

Yes, a *lot* of years to go. I always wanted to turn 40. I don't know why. [Older women] are sexy, and they've lived, and yet there's so much more life to live. I think 40 is like the best age for a woman. My mom, when she was 40 … she was gorgeous. Maybe that's why.

Do you look like your mom?

You know, everybody says I look more like my father.

He's a beautiful man. *(Laughs)*

Yes, he is.

Is there anything you'd like to add?

For people to take care of their health, because if you're healthy, you're going to look better. And to exercise, even though you don't like it. I don't like doing exercises, but I know that I have to do them. Thirty minutes of cardio every day. So eat well, sleep well, and go to the gym.

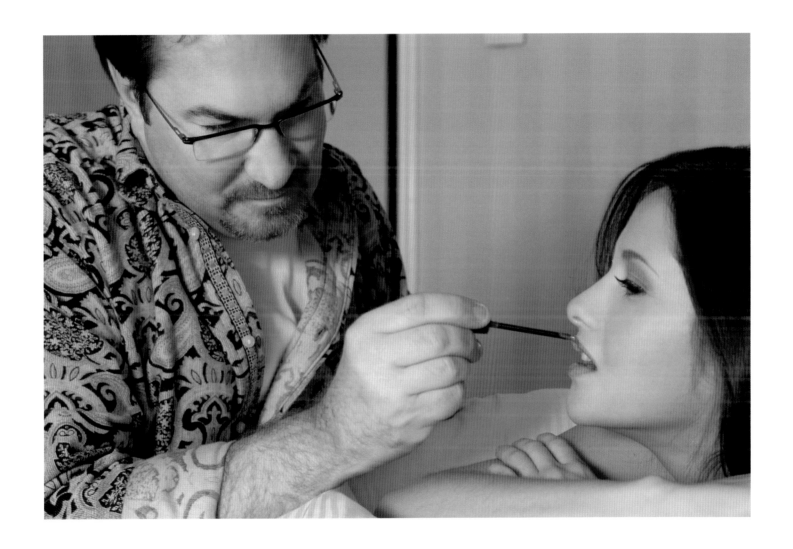

FARAH FATH

As far as I can tell, Farah Fath has always known she had "it"—you know, that magical, intangible quality that Simon Cowell is always going on and on about on *American Idol*. She's lovely, for starters. And she isn't merely luminous, she's bright—a big distinction in Hollywood. So it isn't a stretch to imagine that when she decided at age 5 to pursue a show-business career, she already had formulated the master plan that would take her from pageants (she was Miss Kentucky Preteen in 1995) to advertisements (Pringles on TV, Duncan Hines in magazines) to daytime TV. Heck, her success in L.A. is the stuff of legend: She'd scarcely unpacked when *Days of Our Lives* offered her the role of mischievous Mimi Lockhart. Of course, her story doesn't end there. Since her 1999 *Days* debut, she's taken her character from smart-mouthed sidekick to heartbreaking heroine, in the process racking up her first primetime credits—on *American Dreams* and *Friends*, no less. Where will the future take this savvy go-getter? My guess is anywhere she damn well pleases. In fact, I'd even put money on it. Lend an ear, won't you, as she sits down with me to discuss everything from make-up to making out.

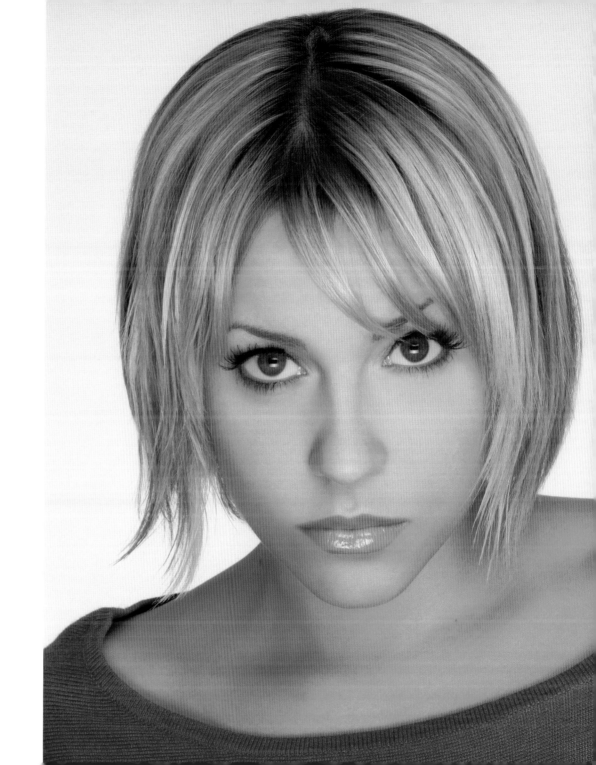

"I LOVE DOING MAKE-UP, WHICH IS AN ART IN ITSELF"

FARAH FATH

Let's start with a little game of compare and contrast. How does your beauty compare to your *Days* character's?

Mimi's beauty is her innocence; she's so naive sometimes. But she knows she's trendy. She does her make-up well, and her hair's funky. My beauty is, I like to wear things that are flattering, and I'll do my make-up natural, and sometimes not, depending on how I'm feeling. We're very similar, obviously, because my attributes are passed on to her.

Hard to believe, given how young you are, but you've been playing Mimi for five years already. Has her look changed in that time?

Like you wouldn't believe. I've probably been through, like, 100 different haircuts and a million different styles. Mimi was always the girl that was trying to fit in, so she would try different looks just to see if she could get attention from guys. I remember there was a hairstyle one time where she had six different ponytails all over her head. I thought that was cool. Then, finally, as she grew up, she felt more comfortable in her own skin and realized that she didn't have to try to be beautiful, because she was.

That's a great metaphor for life—you search and search until you realize you had what you were searching for all along. Do you have a guilty pleasure?

I get massages all the time. I just read in a magazine that the third most important thing besides eating healthy and exercise is touch, like getting a massage. I totally believe it. If you get all that lactic acid build-up out of there, your body just looks and feels better.

From whom do you take your beauty cues? Mom? Magazines? Make-up artists?

As far as trends go, I've learned so much just by being in Hollywood. I'm from Kentucky, so I see such a difference from Southern or Midwestern states. They get all the trends like two years later. I was just there last week, and girls were just starting to wear pointy shoes. I was like, "I was wearing those three years ago." And they're just starting to get layers in their hair. It's really wild the way the country is.

And people think there's only a *political* divide. Ha! Do you have a favorite leading man?

The guy who plays my boyfriend, Rex. His name is Eric Winter. He's my best friend in real life. He's the guy in the new Britney Spears commercial [for her fragrance, Curious]. He's gorgeous—inside, too. I've been lucky enough to get to know him really well. He's a total sweetheart.

Aside from Eric, what actor would you *like* to have a sexy screen moment with?

Obviously, it's a toss-up between Brad Pitt and Orlando Bloom. Let's go with Brad. How many people have picked him?

Nobody. But I've gotten a George Clooney. Do you feel like soap stars get the credit they deserve from the mainstream press?

No. We work harder than any other actor out there. I mean, I've had 90 pages in one night to memorize, and I don't see ...

... someone off camera calling out your lines to you!

No. We've got huge fan bases, yet if I go to an award show and there are primetime people there or music stars, it's as if I'm just a regular person. It doesn't even matter. And that's fine, but at least personally, if I ever move on to do film or whatever, I will have the greatest appreciation for daytime dramas and all the people who work on them.

Do you have any hidden talents that your fans might not know about? And no, that's not a dirty question.

I paint. I like acrylics.

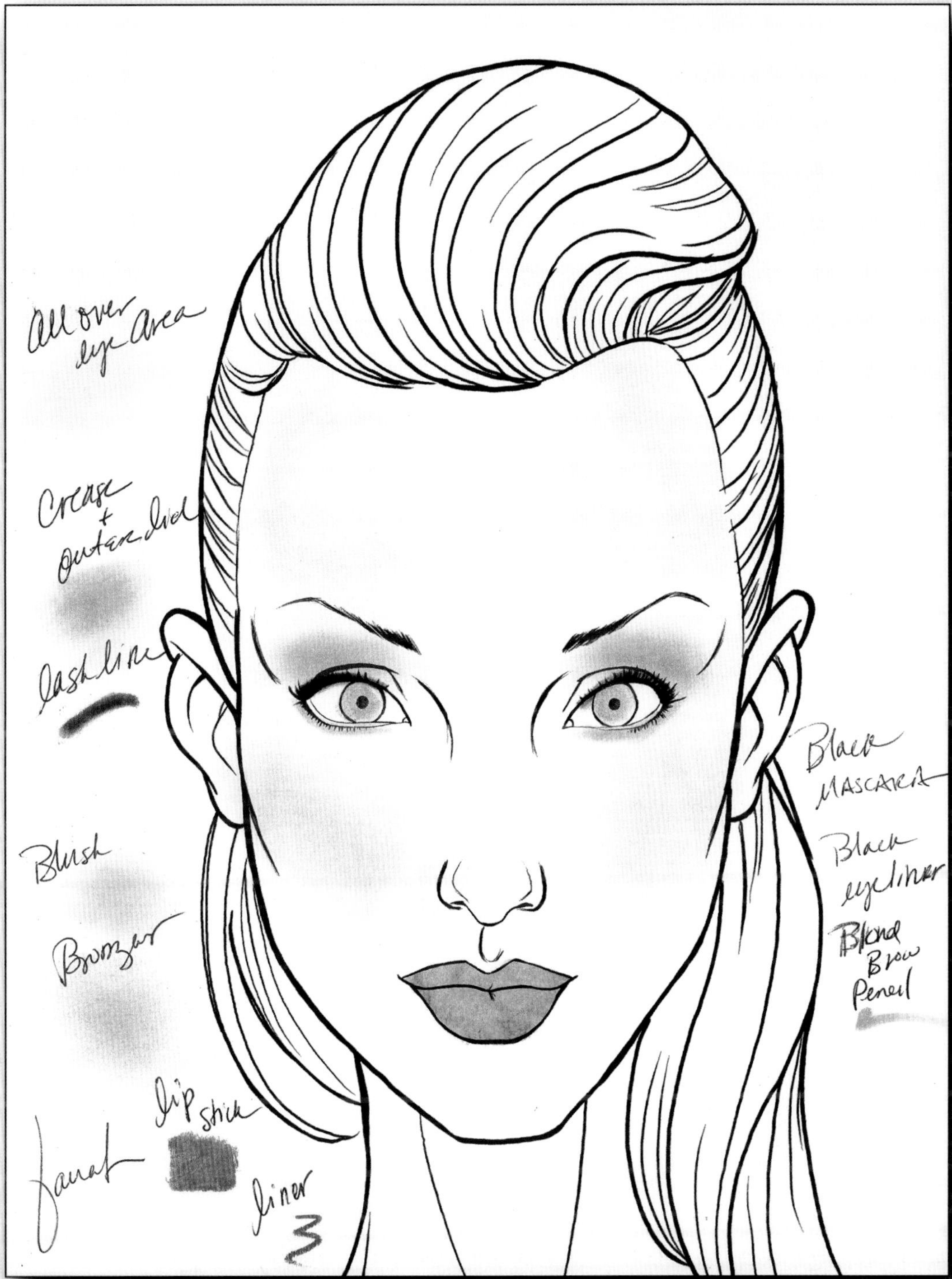

All over eye area

Crease + outer lid

lash line

Blush

Bronzer

Black MASCARA

Black eyeliner

Blond Brow Pencil

lip stick

liner 3

Have you ever had a show?

No. I never felt like my stuff was good enough. But then, people will look at it and go, "That's awesome! Who did this?" and I'll go, "Eh, that was me." I don't get all artsy-fartsy, but I love doing make-up, which is an art in itself. I love putting together outfits, and that in itself is an art. Painting and decorating my house … that's what I love to do.

When you need to replenish your strength, where do you turn?

I call my little sister, as weird as that sounds.

I only think that's weird if you're a member of the Hilton family.

My sister's 17, but if I'm ever having a problem, she's the first person I call. Her name's Victoria. She gives good advice. I just feel most comfortable telling her most anything and everything.

Let's see how comfortable you are doing the same with me. What's your biggest turn-on in a guy?

Sense of humor. I'm a pretty funny person, so I need someone that can be right at that level with me. I've never been so much about looks. He's just gotta make me laugh and treat me with respect. That's it.

Biggest turn-off?

B.O. and dirty fingernails. I dated a guy who had dirty fingernails, and it's really like, "Do I want you touching me with those hands? No. So clean your fingernails and put deodorant on!"

This may be an interesting question for you since you're so young. Is there anything missing from the world now that you once enjoyed?

I want to say innocence, but that's not really the word. When you're younger, you don't know what's out there. You just know that you've got your mom, you've got your dad, you've got your sucker, and you're ready to go. This past week-end, I was in Miami and I got to party with some high-profile Hollywood stars and got to see for the first time the bad side of Hollywood. I've lived out here for five years and didn't really think that sort of thing went on, but it does, and it's a shame. So, now I got to see it, and I know that I will never fall into that.

I don't think you will, either. You're too smart for that.

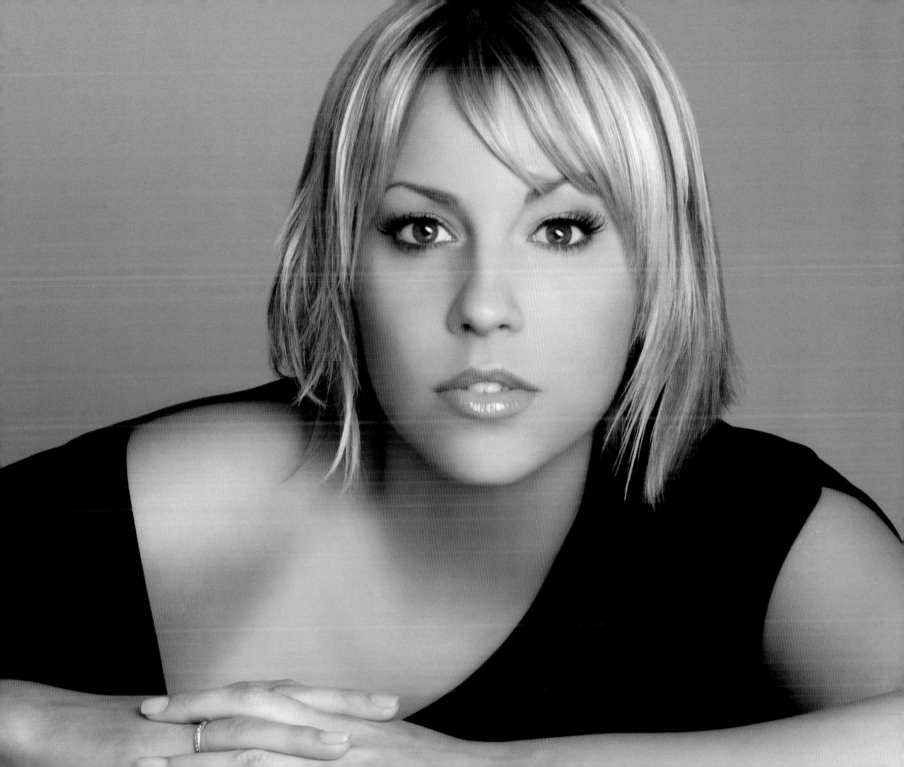

CHAPTER 5:

Base Instincts

"It makes me feel older!" "It makes me feel like I'm wearing a mask!" "I hate it, I hate it, I hate it!"

No, ladies, these are not quotes that I have gotten from actresses who have had to lock lips with a bad love-scene partner. These are remarks I have heard from everyday women regarding foundation. (While many a celebrity make-up artist gives up his or her ordinary clientele, I never have—I still do proms, weddings, divorces … you name it. Guess I'm a sucker for milestones. But I digress …) I swear, if I had a powder puff for every complaint I've heard about foundation, I could talc the tush of the world!

However, there is no need for all this negativity. Foundation can be the—all together now—*foundation* of a beautiful make-up job. You need only keep in mind your skin type: Is it oily? Dry? Some combination of the two that you are sure is found on no other face on the planet? How you answer is critical, so be honest

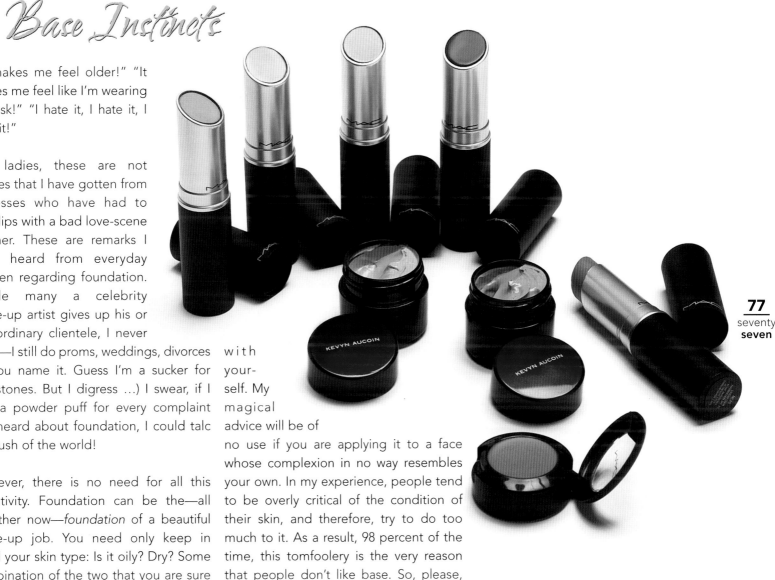

with yourself. My magical advice will be of no use if you are applying it to a face whose complexion in no way resembles your own. In my experience, people tend to be overly critical of the condition of their skin, and therefore, try to do too much to it. As a result, 98 percent of the time, this tomfoolery is the very reason that people don't like base. So, please, help me help you by facing facts—even if the facts aren't so good. Okay?

Now let's look at some of the many and varied formulas from which you could select your base. (I know: It's intimidating. But after some trial and error, you're going to play favorites with the formula you like best, and you can avoid this hazard for life. Or at least a really, really long time.)

FIRST UP

Liquid base (and all its permutations). Not to be confused with Ace of Base. (And certainly not to be confused with Asa Buchanan.) Usually a light to medium liquid, sometimes with SPF.

Cream foundation, which is usually heavier and best reserved for drier complexions; gives flawless coverage.

Tinted moisturizer, which is so sheer that it offers no coverage at all; on the plus side, it usually comes anywhere between SPF 8 and SPF 15.

Mineral base, which is great for sensitive skin and those of you who are skittish. (Skittish people rarely get enough vitamins and minerals, you see. Kidding.)

Dual finish base, whose name says it all.

Ah ah ah! No freaking out yet. (Save that for your next brow wax.) I'm not done yet. If you like a light base, a water-based liquid foundation is perfect for you. Are you a teenager? (Again, be honest!) Then, a tinted moisturizer would be great to protect and even out your skin tone. For those of you whose complexion brings to mind the Sahara, the use of a moisturizing liquid should be such a no-brainer that you'll have plenty of gray matter left to choose between brands. I like a stick and cream base for dehydrated skin, an evening look or any time that heavier coverage is needed. But, while you and I are both here in these parentheses, let me remind you that it would be unwise to try to get your skincare from make-up. If you've read the "Saving Face" chapter—and if you haven't, for shame!—you can pretty much use a basic liquid, as your skin will be balanced and the moisture barrier already established.

When in doubt at all, pay a visit to a professional. If you can't admit that you are in doubt, and won't let me give you the number of a good therapist, at least refrain from choosing a base by holding the cardboard shade up to your face. And for the love of God, don't ever hold the cardboard up to your hand! I've seen that done in supermarkets, drug stores … anywhere that testers are not available, and it kills me every time! My stance is, if you can't try it (on your face!), you shouldn't buy it (period). So, if the sales clerk doesn't or won't open a tester and show you where and how to test it, move on, fast.

I've *been* a counter person, and I know: This is what we are paid to do (and if we're any good at it at all, we want to make sure you get the right stuff, not just a lot of stuff).

That brings us to application. Convenient, no? I like to apply base by putting some on the back of my hand, then filling a sponge with it by wiping it into the sponge. Then, in essence, I wash the face with it, starting at the center and working my way out, blending as I go. (This way, you use less product and get a more natural look.)

Side note: Here is something that I always do that some people adore, others abhor. So, I'll tell you about it, and you can decide for yourself whether it's something you'd like to try. Here goes: I always put foundation on first and then concealer on *top* unless the individual on whom I am working has major areas of concern (in which case I put it on both sides, lightly). Why do I do this? As a person who lives in the real world, your objective should be to use as little make-up as possible to achieve the look that you want. And most of the time, foundation covers the light discoloration you may see on your face; thus, it takes less make-up to make it up and disappear. Got it? Now then, on to concealer! How do I love this product? Let me count the ways! I love it because it brings light to the face. I love it because it

brings coverage to areas of concern. I love it because …

Okay, so I only love it two ways. But you have to admit: They're *good* ways.

As do most make-ups, concealer comes in several packaging types. But—you'll like this, I am confident—we are only going to discuss one. Uno. Singular. And the winner is … concealer in a pot! Which is actually not so much a pot as it is a little jar. (A little jar of beauty, if you will.) When using this product, you are actually going to use less of it, because it is heavier and covers better. (Seeing exactly how much you are doling out of the pot doesn't hurt, either.)

To apply, use a concealer brush to softly paint small layers on your areas of concern. If more concealer is needed, use a little more. (If you're on the fence, quit while you're ahead—the finished product will be much more natural-looking.)

With regard to concealer, my biggest area of concern—philosophically speaking, not facially—is you women who purchase concealer in wands or lipstick tubes, and think about it mainly in the morning. Why would you do that? I beseech you: Don't! When you apply tube concealer before your first cup of coffee, you are tired and, for all practical purposes, rolling the product around on your face until you have erased every expression you ever had. That is not the point of this product. (Doing away with your emotions is the point of botox and gin. But that's another story altogether.) As far as color goes, I recommend using a concealer that is a shade lighter than your foundation, which, if you have been paying attention, will be the same shade as the skin on your face, not on cardboard. (Remember?)

Finally, we are ready to take a powder. By which I mean that we are ready to discuss powder. A lot of people skip it. "It makes my skin look old," they whine. Or they say, "I just can't figure it out," and give up trying. But really, this is an easy one. If you have on a foundation and concealer, you need powder to *set* them. If the foundation and concealer aren't set, they will move as your body temperature rises and drops—and yes, that can be as grody as it sounds. It can even affect your skin texture! (Once more, with feeling: Ew!) So, for your own good, get powdered.

The best is an invisible powder to set your foundation—preferably a loose powder, which you can then press to set with a sponge or puff. (Once you've set your product, it ain't goin' nowhere! At least not until you remove it yourself.) Pressed powder, on the other hand, is great for a quick touch-up on the road; it's also aces if you are on a fixed budget. Any other kind of powder is just for fun—those occasions when you want to not only glow but shimmer, bronze, etc.

And just like that, I've got you, ahem, covered.

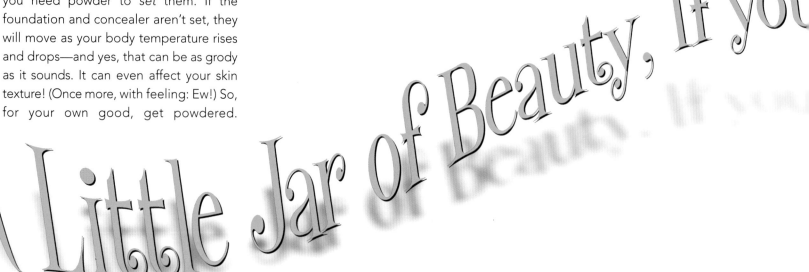

A Little Jar of Beauty, If you

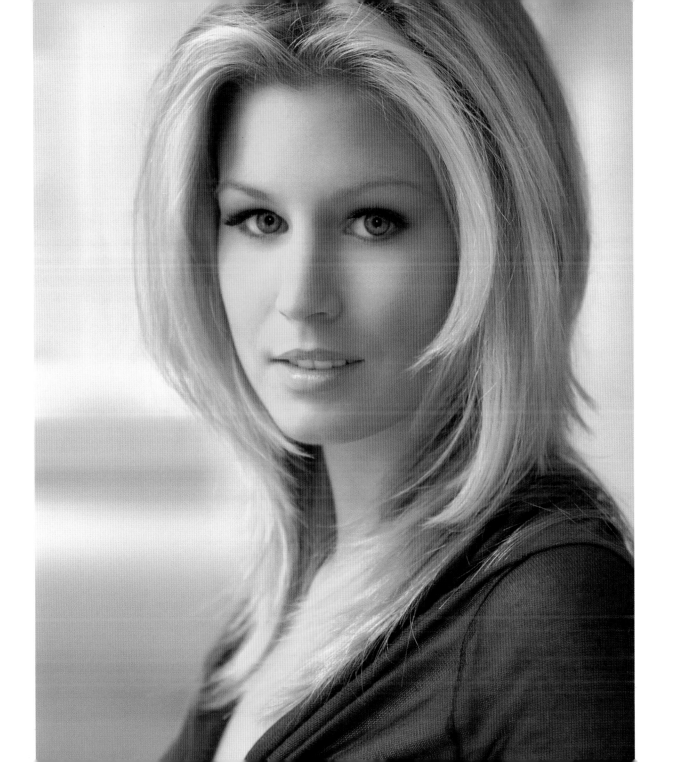

will

ROBIN MATTSON

Robin Mattson once said to me, "You're family." And when I'm with her, I certainly do feel that way. Before we met more than a decade ago, the grownup child star was already well-established in showbiz, thanks to her guest appearances on *Flipper*, *Charlie's Angels* and damn near every series in between. She'd also conquered daytime television, quickly giving up playing ho-hum heroines (like *Guiding Light*'s Hope Bauer) to enliven villainesses with va-va-voom (among them, *General Hospital*'s Heather Webber and *Santa Barbara*'s Gina Capwell). When we finally hooked up—not like *that*—she was stirring the pot on *All My Children* as ex-con Janet "From Another Planet" Green. But I would soon learn that there was little, if anything, that the native Californian couldn't do if she set her mind to it. For instance: She loves food. Cooking. Dining. All of it. So she studied her butt off, became a chef whose name alone makes her friends salivate, wrote a cookbook (*Soap Opera Café: The Skinny on Food From a Daytime Star*) and finally went all Julia Child as host of *The Main Ingredient*. Needless to say, our "family" dinners have been scrumptious! Today probably isn't the day that you'll join us for a snack, but perhaps you'll enjoy these excerpts from our conversation, anyway. In a manner of speaking, they, too, are food … for thought.

"IT'S
FUN
TO
BE
EXTREME"

ROBIN MATTSON

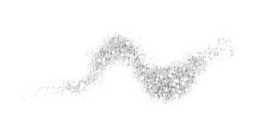

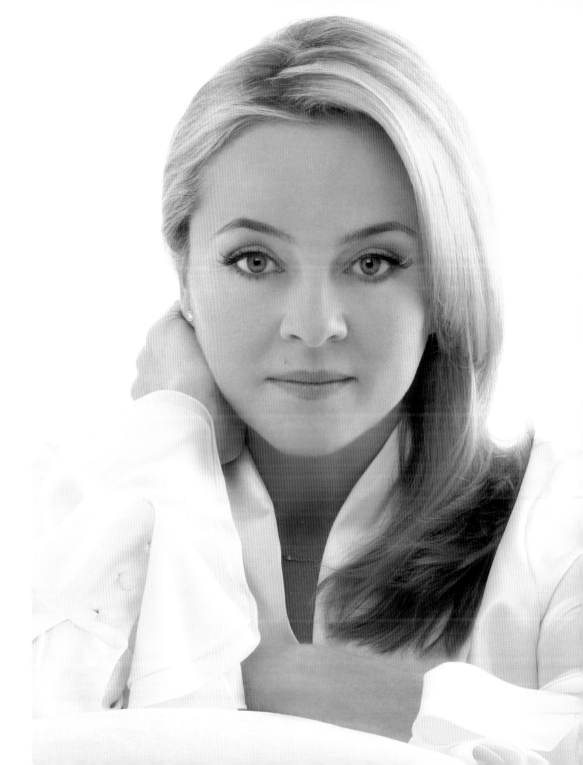

What is your take on beauty?

Oh, it's so individual and so varied. It's incredible how one person will see something one way, and another person will be like, "No. I just don't get it. What are you talking about?" It's truly in the eye of the beholder. I mean, I definitely have an idea of what I think is beautiful. You can see someone beautiful across the room, and somehow, they're just not pretty, and I don't want to know them. That sounds really judgmental, but it's true. There is something that exudes from the person.

B.O., usually. *(Laughs)* I'm kidding. Something does resonate from people.

No matter how they look on the outside. [Something] makes you want to know them, get close to them—or keep your distance.

What would you say your personal style is?

Probably a little more conservative than I like, not so much in personality, but ...

Classic.

Classic. I like that.

Whenever we've shot together, I've thought that: You're classically stunning.

Well, thank you. A general motto is, "Always be overdressed rather than underdressed." I don't like to feel that I'm not appreciative or respectful of a situation because I'm underdressed, as I am today. *(Laughs)* I told you before I came over [to do the shoot], "I look junky." I figured you'd probably just be in jeans.

Honey, you make even jeans look like haute couture. Relax. Now tell me, do you have a real-life make-up horror story? I don't want to answer the question for you, but I always remember the story about you in Russia and the guy who was reusing dirty sponges on you.

Ah, yes, that was me. And then they did another crazy thing—they sprayed the make-up on.

Like airbrushing?

They airbrushed on the make-up. I thought, "These are crazy people. These are techniques that I don't know if they're cutting-edge, but they're certainly unique."

Robert [Milazzo, the photographer] bought the machine!

(Laughs, then simulates the sound of spray-painting) Sssssst!

We tried it out on a model, but I was appalled, because every time I would spray her, she would pull her face back. I need more control than that offers, anyway.

It's kind of a new nightmare in each city. I had one guy pull out a bunch of dirty sponges and old make-up. You know when lipstick gets that smell … when it's rancid?

Oh, yeah. Some of my favorite colors stink now. It's tragic! *(Laughs)* Moving on, do you have a best make-up story?

I think I was talking to [my fiancé] about what makes a photograph come together, and I said what I was feeling in terms of both you and Robert is some familiarity. You know your subject. You know what works. It's hard to do your best work the first time you're shooting someone or your first time doing someone's hair and make-up. Familiarity breeds excellence.

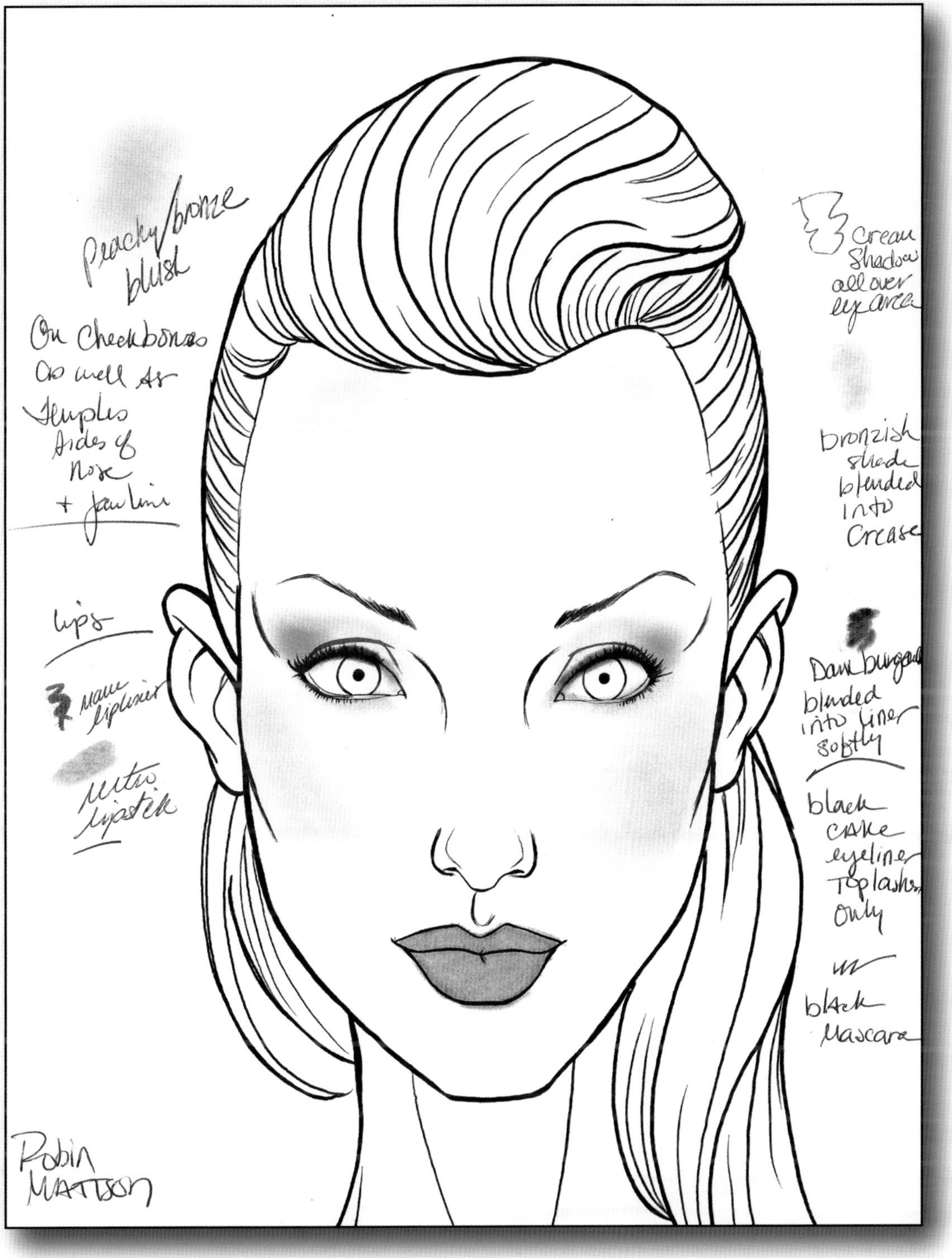

Peachy/bronze blush

On cheekbones as well as temples sides of nose + jawline

lips

mauve lipliner

netro lipstick

cream shadow all over eye area

bronzish shade blended into crease

Dark burgundy blended into liner softly

black cake eyeliner top lashes only

black mascara

Robin MATTSON

It's trust, too. How many times have I done your make-up and you've turned around and said, "Be a blender." Or, "Tim, more eye cream." Or you'll be chasing me for more moisturizer. These are things that I love about working on you, not just because they're amusing, but because they represent a level of trust. I've always trusted you enough that you'd say to me, "Tim, I need more" or "I want less" …

… rather than go in the next room and say, "Oh my God, what has this man just done to me?!"

Speaking of villainy, that's been your niche on soaps. Don't you ever want to play the nice lady with three kids who stays home and bakes after sending her honey off to work?

Originally, Hope Bauer on *Guiding Light* was very pure.

But once you got there … !

No, she was the ingenue, the girl next door. That's why when I went in to audition for *General Hospital* [to play Heather, the loco character originated by Cher's sister, Georganne LaPiere], I thought they'd never cast me, because my one and only role on daytime was as this ingenue. But I guess somebody saw something in me.

Well, you *are* intense. In a good way. *(Laughs)*

What you do is, you grab up this intensity from within you, and you exaggerate it and turn it into extreme acting.

I love that whenever I hear people talk about you and your characters, they talk about how bad they are!

It's fun to be bad, and it's fun to be extreme. I'm kind of an over-the-top person myself, not in the way my characters are, but I feel things extremely. I'm emotional, so I can usually take [my emotions] wherever the character is going.

Is there anything missing in the world today that you once had that is no more?

Well, my first thought is my father, but we all have people that we love that we miss. I went to culinary school after he passed away, and [that career] was all sort of a tribute to him, and it was a creative desire that I had to pursue that came from him. But I wish so much that I could share that with him, to have him see me graduate from culinary school, to see the cookbook …

Is there another book in you? *(Long pause)* There is! I think there is!

There are so many cookbooks on the market that it's hard to come up with something new and different with a commercial angle that will sell well.

If anybody can do it, I'd put my money on that person being you. So what *are* your plans now that Heather's back in the loony bin? What's going on?

Well, I'm in love. I'm happy. I found someone who's a wonderful partner. We're a good team, working together, slaying the dragons. It's nice to have someone say that it's not the end of the world and it's not about you. It's wonderful to find the person you feel you want to get old with and spend the rest of your life with.

JADE HARLOW

Jade Harlow is a modern girl through and through. So young and full of life is she that she isn't so much "today" as she is "tomorrow." Yet her favorite films include two old Bette Davis classics, *Hush, Hush, Sweet Charlotte* and *Whatever Happened to Baby Jane?* Which is the real Harlow? Both. And that's why I am confident that she will someday see her own name in lights. Obviously, she's gorgeous; Noxzema couldn't conceivably find a fresher-faced spokesperson. Certainly, she's charismatic; as *Passions* plaything Jessica Bennett, the luminous newcomer did as much to light the set as any crew member. But moreover, she is a classic. In Hollywood's Golden Age, she would have been signed to a studio and given free rein to take any and every ingenue part there was to be had. The Vegas native knows how (and when) to gamble, too: During our shoot, she was up for anything, and the results speak for themselves. She knows who (and when) to trust, and in any instance of doubt, relies on instincts that belie her tender age. So I say, "Enjoy your 15 minutes of fame while they last, Natalie Portman; Jade Harlow is comin' for ya!" Here's the interview that proves I knew her when …

"...GET BACK DOWN TO THE SIMPLE ELEMENTS"

JADE HARLOW

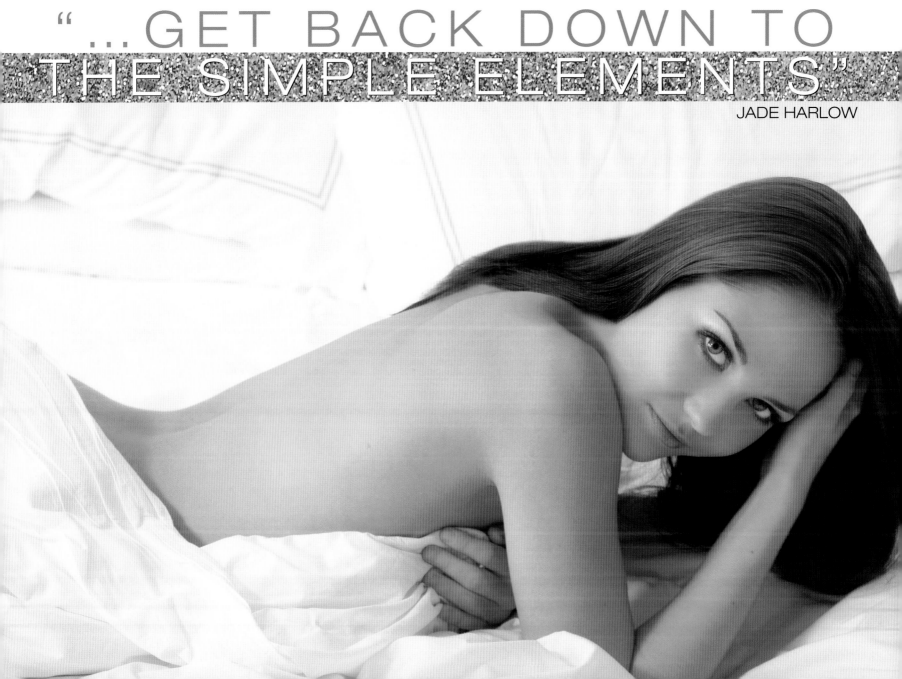

Are you anything like your *Passions* character?
When I started playing Jessica, I wasn't as nice as I am now that I've played such a good person for so long. It actually made me a better, more empathetic person.

I'm afraid to ask—what were you like before?
I was kind of a bitch.

Really? You were one of the *Mean Girls*?
You know, when you're not real popular in school, you get that chip on your shoulder, and you just kind of carry it around. That was me when I started working on *Passions*.

Was the soap your big break?
No. I did some stuff before. I did a stint on *Third Rock from the Sun*, and I did an independent film where I played Priscilla Presley.

No kidding! Who played Elvis?
Peter Dobson. He did a show on USA called *FBI Family*.

So, at 21 years old, what is your take on beauty?
I love old Hollywood glamour. I think there's a big difference between that and what is glamorous nowadays. I kind of feel the pressure to compete with girls my age who are going out and getting surgery. I could name names, but I mean, it's pretty obvious who's doing it. So I feel like I have to get that eventually. But when you look at the classic beauties— Vivien Leigh, for example—you don't need it. I think that, in the short and long term, is more beautiful than this new glamour where [actresses will] show as much skin as they can.

It scares me sometimes, how far people go with plastic surgery.
So many people start to look exactly alike—you know, the fake tan, the bleached teeth, the blond hair, the big boobs. It's like there's no individuality when it comes to beauty. And then you look at people like Angelina Jolie or Natalie Wood, who to me is another classic beauty. I wish everything would get back to that.

People always laugh at me, but I still say that Barbra Streisand is a beautiful woman.
(Laughs)

See?!
Her eyes are magnificent.

Yes! And she was her own character; she walked around with such pride.
That comes from a feeling inside.

I would think so. But I digress. Let's talk about you. What is your personal style?
Day to day, it's the alternative look. I like a pair of fitted jeans, a cool band T-shirt with a neat neckline. I like to take T-shirts and make my own necklines. I love vintage jackets. A jacket and a belt to me can make any outfit.

Where beauty's concerned, what do you think you have to hide, if anything?
Or are you pretty much a take me-as-I-am girl?
I'm too self-conscious to be take-me-as-I-am, but what I would like to hide is the lack of confidence. I paint confidence on with my make-up. It makes me feel better, and it doesn't have to be gobs of make-up, just an evened-out skin tone, stuff like that. If I wanted to hide any physical flaw, I have a scar from a dog bite. That's pretty much it.

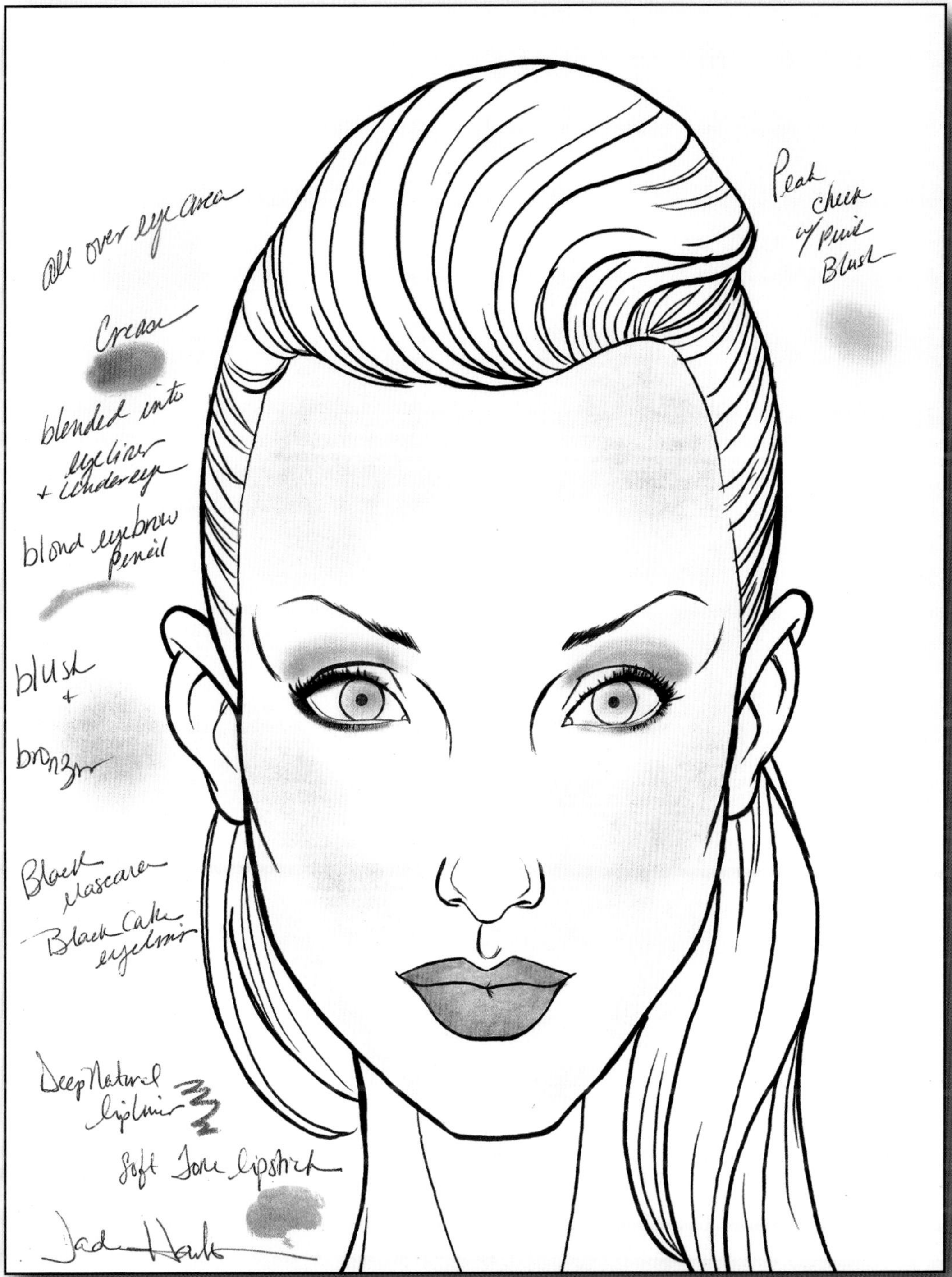

All over eye area

Crease

blended into
eye liner
+ under eye

blond eyebrow
pencil

blush
+

bronzer

Black
Mascara

Black Cake
eyeliner

Deep Natural
lipliner

Soft Tone lipstick

Peak
cheek
w/ pink
Blush

I can't believe you don't just walk into a room and say, "Here I am." I pegged you as having confidence, just not the manic, in-your-face kind. It's like you're 21 going on 40.

That's what I feel like.

You seem to have a quiet core.

Why, thank you. I think that quiet core helps when you walk into a room with beautiful women who have done so much to tweak their appearance to be the socialized ideal of perfection. You do feel the pressure to compete. I'm pretty confident when it comes to my personality and being able to wow a room with my quick wit and intelligence, but walking into a room and wowing them with my looks, that's a lot of pressure. I feel I have to paint something on to help out a little bit.

I get by with a little help from my friends, base and concealer, too. Do you have a make-up horror story?

Oh, yeah, because I've experimented with everything that's ever come out. There was this make-up for stars that was supposed to make your skin beautiful, but it was a big flop. I put this crap on my face, and it must have taken me a week to get it off. Every time I sweat, it would come out of my pores, and it was like wax. It caused a lot of bad breakouts.

Do you believe that make-up has power?

To an extent, yes. Whatever is inside, whether it be good, bad or ugly, is going to radiate no matter how much you put on or alter your appearance. If you're an ugly human being at heart, you're going to be an ugly human being no matter what you do to yourself. But I think that if you're shy and not too confident, but you know that you've got good things going for you, a little bit of make-up can help you be yourself in front of a room full of people.

It's almost unfair of me to ask this of a 21-year-old, but what's the hardest lesson you've learned so far?

The friends situation. I wasn't really popular in school, but when I came out here and started working on Passions, it's like there's this money and you have these friends and you want everyone to be around you, so you buy them things. I ended up, when all was said and done, not having anybody who was worth anything. So I've learned that if you can be an a—hole and those friends still stick around, those are the real friends.

You really impress me. You've got your head screwed on straight. Any parting words?

I just think it's a great idea what you're doing with the book. Women feel a lot of pressure with this new beauty going on, and so let's just try to get back down to the simple elements to show that that's all you need.

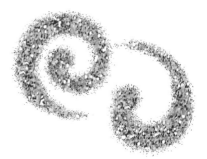

CHAPTER 6:

Feeling Cheeky

Remember how I told you that make-up wasn't rocket science? Well, the makers of blush would like nothing better than to convince you otherwise. That's why they turn out their product in as many formulas as there are *reasons* to go red-faced, and create the stuff in powder form, cream form, bronzing form, cheek-staining-stick form…

Confused yet? Lord knows, these companies want you to be. As long as they can keep you overwhelmed, they can keep you, period—coming back season after season, only to be given the same advice as last time … which, not coincidentally, sets you up to return again in three months to restart the cycle. But—aha!—with a little of your time and my guidance, we can change that.

First things first: What, exactly, *is* blush? According to *Funk & Wagnalls* (and who doesn't prefer a dictionary with funk right there in the title?), it's "a red or rosy tint." The made-up version of blush is pretty much the same thing: a bit of color applied to your cheek, just to make you feel a little brighter or livelier on those deadly dull gray days. (Okay, so *Funk & Wagnalls* didn't say anything about raising

your spirits; I'm sure it was an oversight.) Imagine the way your cheeks look when you've just come in from a blustery December day—that's blush. Anything above or beyond that is purely paint. Not that there's anything wrong with that. It just bore mentioning.

The next big issue that arises when discussing blush is, "Where the hell does it go?" Some of you may have a tough time finding your cheekbones (they're there, I assure you). Others may complain that, because you have a round face, you *have* no cheekbones (you do, I again assure you). Still others may lament that your blush never comes out right (it will, just wait). So let's address those concerns, and fast. A good and easy way to locate your cheek-bones is to smile. By doing so, you have inadvertently located your cheeks. Ta-da! (Tough, wasn't it?) If you are still unsure, look in the mirror first thing in the morning, pre-make-up. (Don't be afraid.) Once you

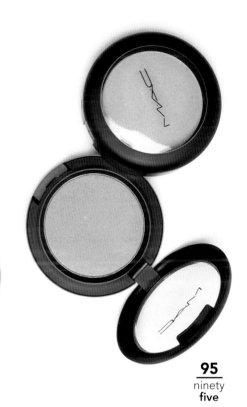

get over the initial shock, touch your cheeks and feel the bone—all the sides of it. While doing so, smile. Ta-da, part deux. C'mon, let's try it right this second, whad'ya say? Take a moment to study your cheeks. I'll wait.

Waiting.

Still waiting.

Okay. Great! See? It's not so hard. You just can't give up; those bones are in there. And once you have nailed this process, you've nailed it for life. (It's not like your cheekbones are going to move.) Then, to achieve a natural look—which I can't recommend highly enough—scoff at the cheek trends that will come down the pike, leaving a trail of clownishly made-up would-be beauties in their wake. Use a soft blush brush to add color high on the cheekbone for day … and slightly lower for evening. It's as quick a pick-me-up as you'll ever need.

Now that we've closed the compact on that dilemma, let's discuss natural selection—that is, the selection of shades that will look natural on you. First, look at your skin tone. (You may wish you had Eva La Rue's mocha coloring or Kassie DePaiva's Georgia-peach complexion, but what you see is what you're stuck with. Not to worry; we'll make it work.) Next, think like Switzerland—in other words, remain neutral. You can *never* go wrong with neutrals, although you should have in your arsenal at least one warm neutral (usually a coral or bronze) and one cool neutral (ordinarily a relative of the pink, mauve or plum families). Fun seasonal shades are just that—fun and seasonal. Much like a summer fling, you really can't count on them beyond the season for which they are designated. (Of course, once in a blue moon, I suppose it's possible that you could fall truly, madly, deeply in love—with a shade, I mean. In which case, buy in bulk, baby, because those time-sensitive hues don't stick around for long. They're like the Cadbury Eggs or Girl Scout cookies of make-up. Mmm …

To do your contouring, you can use a blush or bronzer, or a darker foundation or powder. (It's the one question to which "Whatever!" is honestly an acceptable

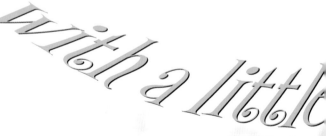

with a little

and appropriate reply.) However, during this process, the application will be a little bit different. For blush, use a darker tone and keep it under the cheek, at the temples and on the sides of the nose. And, by all means, be careful! If those last two words frighten you, then don't contour at all, and especially not during the day; a morning misstep can leave you looking like you're wearing dirt until you notice. You have some more leeway after dark, when, for instance, soft restaurant lighting can enhance the illusion you are trying to put over. See what I mean?

These days, most make-up artists have struck contouring from their repertoires of quick fixes. But, although I use the technique sparingly, and then only to soften a nose or round out a cheek, I still like it. After all, how can it be wrong when it looks so right? So, go ahead and do some experimenting. Then turn the other cheek and watch yourself blush the old-fashioned way when you see how hot you look!

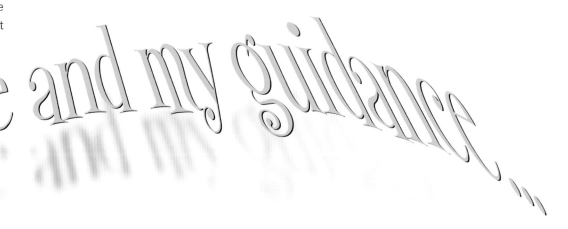
of your time and my guidance

EVA LA RUE

Eva La Rue isn't just a soap actress, she is a true soap *star*. So she could probably get away with pulling diva trips if she wanted to. She could show up late, make demands, be as difficult as she likes. But she never has and never would, and that, my friends— forgetting all about her perfect, caramel complexion and big, Bambi-esque eyes—is why I so adore her. Chances are, it is a good part of the reason you like her, too. Even in her first, brief daytime role, as con artist Margot Collins on *Santa Barbara*, her innate sweetness shone through. (Perhaps that's why the character wasn't a snug fit; who would Eva La Rue ever have to con? People would line up to *give* her what she needs!) In 1993, she struck pay dirt when *All My Children* cast her in a role closer to her own personality: Maria Santos, the brain surgeon with a heart of gold. Since then, she's done everything from primetime hits (among them *Soul Food* and *Third Watch*) to reality television (hosting *Candid Camera* with Dom DeLuise), and worked opposite some of the hottest leading men in creation (*Melrose Place* alum Grant Show, anyone? Eddie Cibrian? Rob Lowe?). With her *AMC* castmate John Callahan, she's also done the most beautiful thing any two people *can* do—brought into the world a baby, their daughter Kaya. If you aren't entirely enamored of the actress-singer-mother-goddess yet, read on. You are gonna fall *so* in love with her.

"BEAUTY IS ALL ABOUT HEALTH AND WHAT THAT ENTAILS"

EVA LA RUE

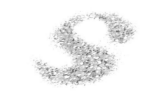

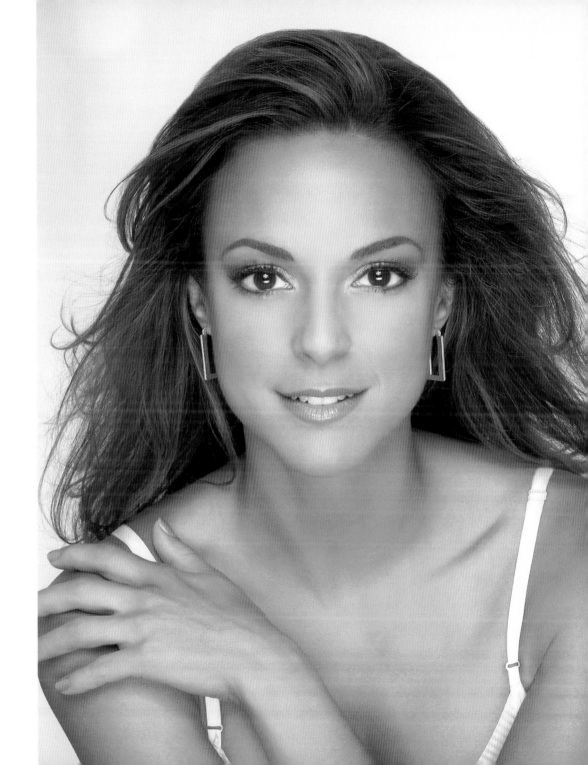

Eva, can you explain to me what your take on beauty is?

Basically, I think beauty is all about health and what that entails—physically, psychologically, internally, externally. When you're totally healthy [and at peace], you're beautiful. And the same goes if somebody is angry or upset … that's not pretty. Sometimes that can be scary! We've all met people like that, and it's unfortunate. Hopefully, they'll find what they are looking for.

We won't mention any names, though. I'll save that for an altogether different book. (Laughs) How long have you been on All My Children now?

I've played Maria for seven years. Well, 11 off and on. I was gone for four.

Has the character's beauty ever changed?

It changed when they brought her back. [When she had amnesia], she was very confused, a very angry woman, and I think she was very ugly then. So I'm glad we're working through that.

Obviously, "ugly" is an exceedingly relative term. What do you think is important for young girls to know about beauty—or the myth of beauty?

It's not something to chase; it's always inside you. It's inside everybody to be the best that they can be.

You weren't in the Army, were you? Just kidding. Was your mother a big influence on you where beauty is concerned?

My mother was the most beautiful woman. She very much reminded me of Marilyn Monroe. She was a single mom, blonde hair, blue eyes, working two, three or four jobs just to keep us kids together.

She definitely made a lasting impression on you, Eva. I've watched your daughter sleep in your arms. That kind of bond, that kind of serenity … it's something to cherish. I had it with my mom, and I suspect you did with yours, too. Before I get all misty, what is the hardest lesson you've ever learned?

That I'm still going through it … that I haven't come out on the other side yet. It's very difficult, but I'll let you know when I get on the other side.

So should I say that this interview is "to be continued"?

Most definitely.

Any last-minute beauty regime that you have to do before you head out the door?

I always put a little powder on my lipstick before I put gloss or anything on. And blot, so it stays on longer. But other than that, I keep it fairly basic.

Do you ever feel insecure about going out in public without any make-up on?

Well, there have been times when I've gone into the grocery store and people have said, "Oh, you look different." You understand that as a celebrity, people watch you all the time, but it makes it difficult to live in the real world. Most people can walk into a grocery without be stared at or followed, or [later] see in the paper that they looked like heck.

I find it hard to believe that you could ever look like heck. C'mon! You are one of my top 10 beauties of all time! That last question I thought was a no-brainer: Your answer should have been no! Seriously, do you think being beautiful has helped you get where you are today?

I'm sure it has, but then again, you see people who are over-polite, and they can advance, too. A lot of times, people will respond to [a good attitude alone] very positively.

Lucky for you, you've got that characteristic in spades as well.

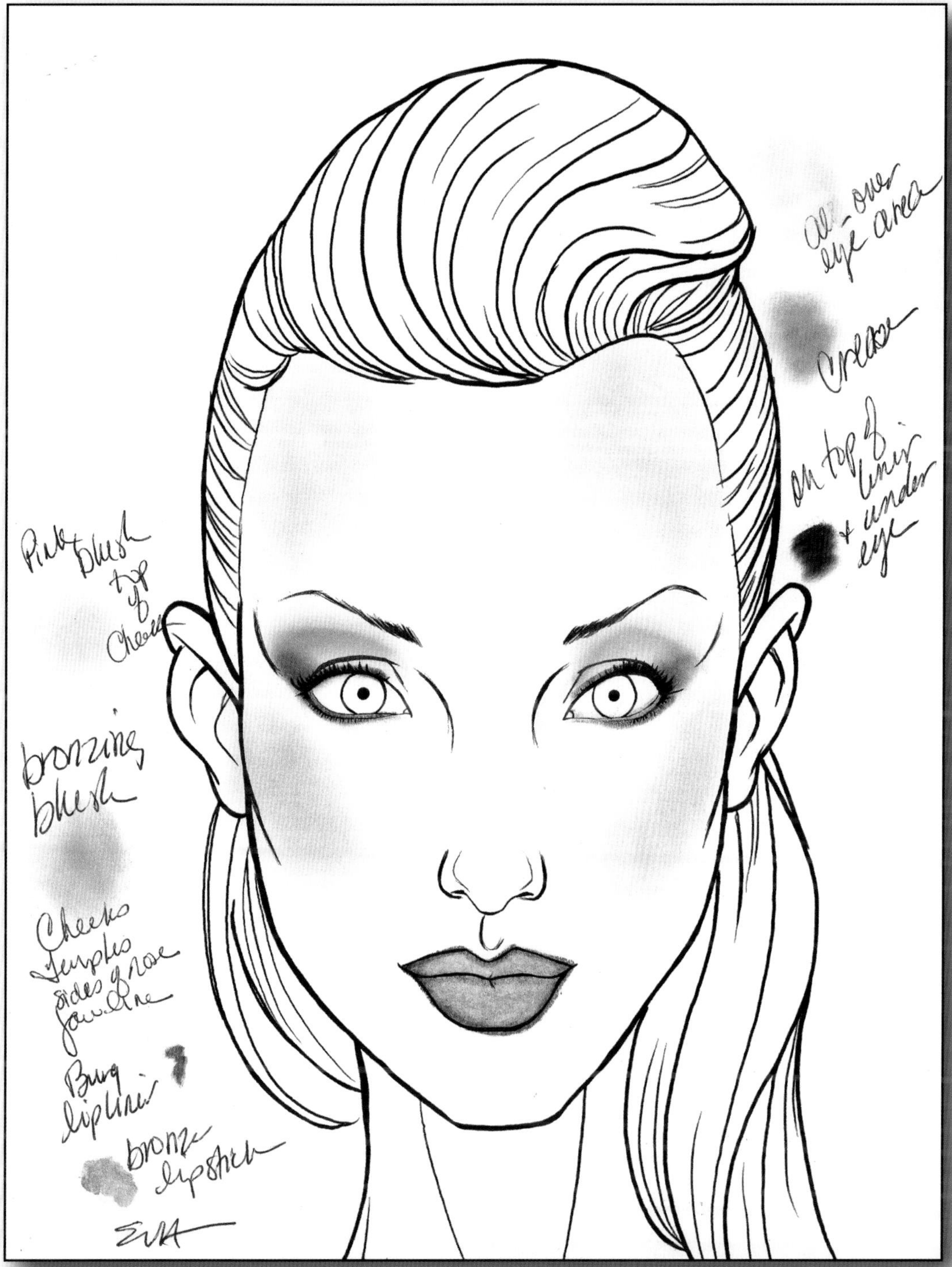

All over eye area

crease

On top of liner + under eye

Pink blush top of cheeks

bronzing blush

Cheeks temples sides of nose jawline

Burg lipliner

bronze lipstick

CRYSTAL CHAPPELL

On screen, Crystal Chappell can fake any quality you want, from coquettishness to dementia. But off screen … uh-uh. Off screen, what she gives you is the real deal, straight up, no chaser. And the real Crystal is *intense*. You can see it in her eyes. Whatever she does, she does with gusto. So it's no wonder she took home a 2002 Emmy for her work as *Guiding Light*'s guileful Olivia Spencer—who but her would have had sharp enough focus to see clear through to the schemer's beating, beaten heart? Thank goodness she gave up her childhood dream of growing up to be a computer geek—that was even her major in college! (Okay, so technically, computer *science* was her major.) But after being cast in a university production of *Beauty and the Beast* (I *know* I don't have to tell you as whom), a star was, if not born, realized. Since being recruited for daytime TV, she has never ceased to challenge herself. First, she made *Days of Our Lives* viewers forget all about supercouple Bo and Hope when, as Dr. Carly Manning, she became Peter Reckell's new leading lady. Next, she had a, um, religious experience, keeping *One Life to Live*'s wannabe nun, Maggie Carpenter, both sassy and soulful. While wowing us, the actress also made an admirer of *Days* castmate Michael Sabatino (who, as Lawrence Alamain, was the third leg of a triangle with Bo and Carly)—to whom she is now wed and has two adorable boys with. Despite the demands of her career and family, she was the first to say, "Just tell me when and where!" when I asked if she would be a part of this book. And, of course, she gave me her full attention during our interview. Go ahead and eavesdrop … you know you want to.

"YOU
CAN
SURPASS
PHYSICAL
BEAUTY,
ALWAYS"

CRYSTAL CHAPPELL

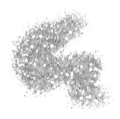

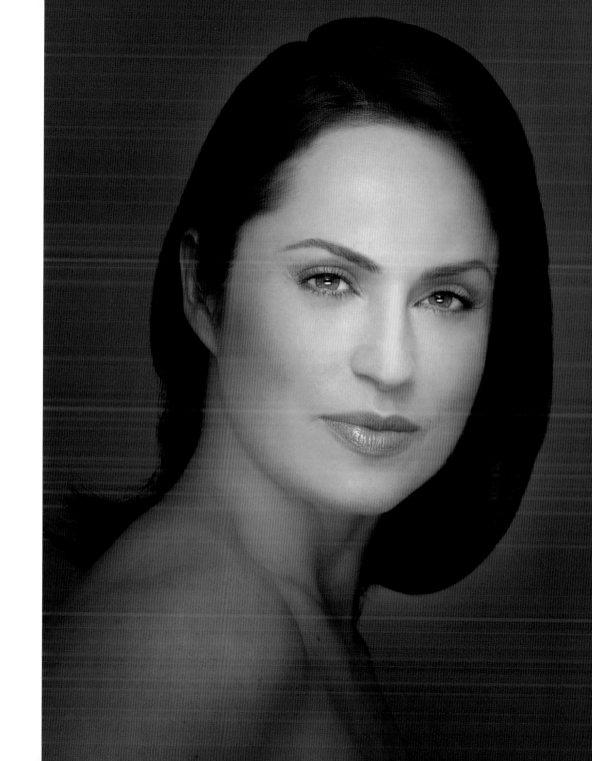

What does beauty mean to you?
There's physical beauty, obviously, but I think what's beautiful is mental spirit and confidence. It's sort of the way I look at life.

Is there a beauty product that you cannot live without?
I use a lot of moisturizer, because I have the driest skin in the world.

Where beauty's concerned, what do you have to hide—or, I should say, "What do you *think* you have to hide?"
I used to feel very uncomfortable with how muscular my body is. Now I'm grateful that I have the strength. When I was a younger woman, it didn't feel feminine to me to have so much muscle, and everyone referred to me as being stocky.

Please! *I'm* stocky; *you're* hot!
(Laughs) Oh, I like your word better.

How do you stay in shape these days? Do you maintain your so-called stockiness just by chasing around the kids?
I really have to work at it, especially now. I like to cross-train, because I get really bored. I like to do interval training on my treadmill … I do yoga and also Pilates once a week. I really like to mix it up, because it works different parts of my body and keeps me interested, which is the main goal for me at this point.

Maybe if I'd ever found doing crunches half as interesting as toffee hazelnut crunch ice cream, I'd look a little more like your leading men. But I digress. Do you believe that make-up has power?
I think so. It depends on a person's taste. I'm always fascinated at the choices women make, what they want to accent.

When do you feel your most beautiful?
First thing in the morning, because I'm in bed with my husband and my two children.

Speaking of your other half, did you two ever keep going on *Days* after the director yelled "Cut!"?
(Laughs) Kissing?

No, playing checkers. Of *course*, kissing!
I don't think so. At least not on the set. Probably after we left the studio, though. He was my first kiss ever as a professional actor.

Boy, did you luck out.
I know. He was a prince.

Now, on *Guiding Light*, you've wound up making out with everybody from Ron Raines (aka Olivia's former sugar daddy, Alan) to Daniel Cosgrove (her boy toy, Bill).
Yeah, I've been around.

Sooo … kiss and tell: Who mouths off the best?
(Laughs) I have to say that they all have their own technique. And I don't want to spill their secrets. I wouldn't kick any of them out.

Aw, chicken. Tell me this, then. As *Days*' Carly, you were buried alive. Are there any beauty secrets for the prematurely interred?
(Laughs) Well, again, it's probably best to stay hydrated. You're going to need that fluid, you know!

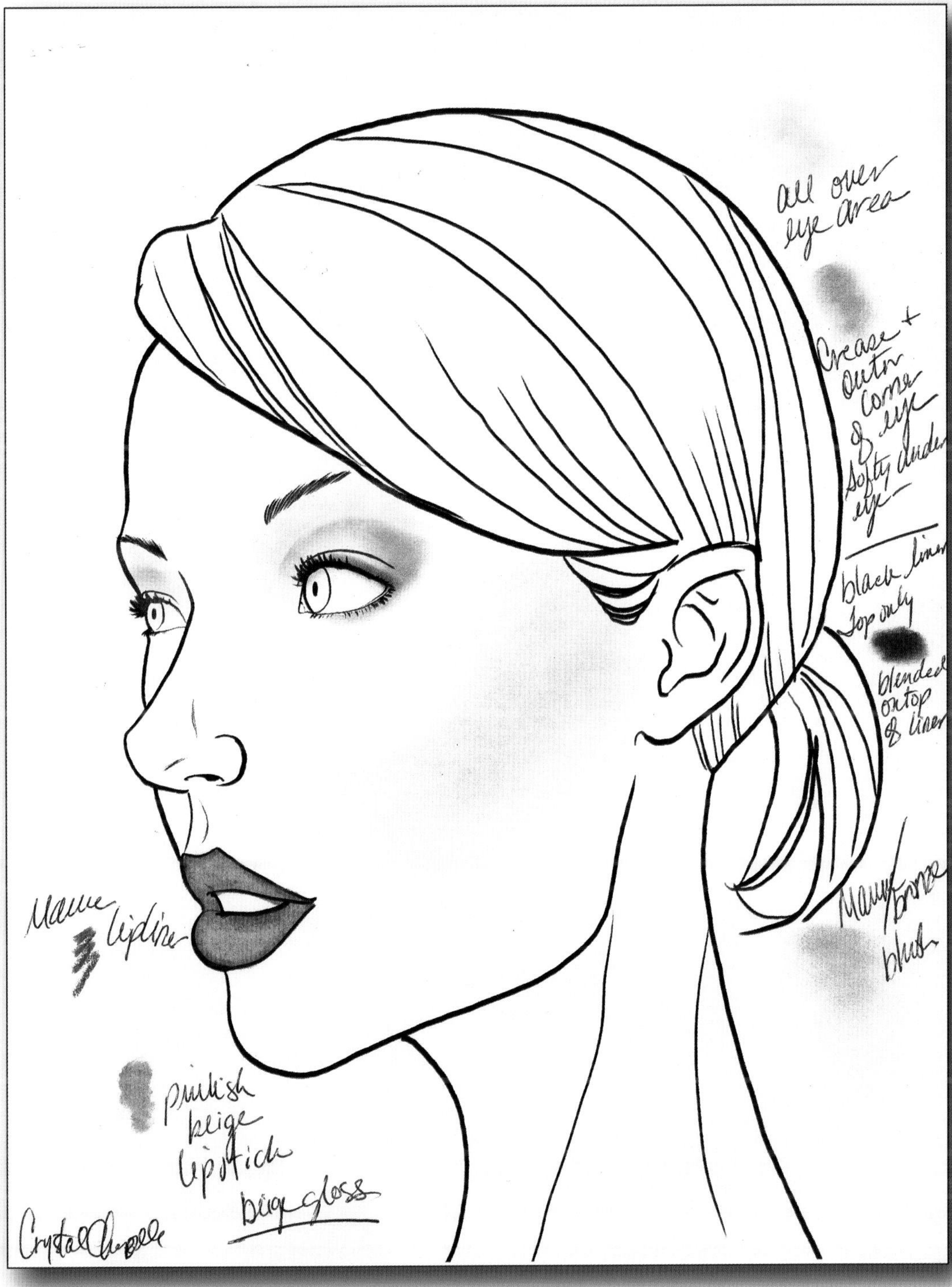

all over
eye area

Crease +
Outer
Corner
of eye
softly under
eye

black liner
top only

blended
on top
of liner

Mauve lipliner

Many bronze
blush

pinkish
beige
lipstick

beige gloss

Crystal Chappell

On a serious note—okay, not *too* serious—do you follow any make-up trends?
Somewhat. To make myself feel better, I've gotten into tanning. Probably once every 10 days. It gives me a little sun-kissed look on my cheek, and I'm fortunate that I have nice enough skin that I don't have to put on foundation with a little bit of color. But I always feel a little naked if I don't have something on my lips. Everything else, I'm okay. Even if it's just a little ChapStick, you know, something. It's like putting on a coat.

When did you realize the power of a woman?
It took me years. When I turned 30, I felt something change in me, and I realized that this was brilliant, with what our bodies do and the power that we have.

That said, what do you think is the most important thing for today's young women to know about beauty?
That you're only as youthful as you feel. And it doesn't really matter what features you're born with, it's what you do with them and how you love yourself. You can surpass physical beauty, always.

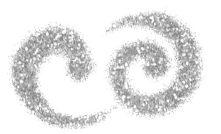

Like you yourself,
your face is a work in progress

CHAPTER 7:

Lip Service

Believe it or not, the farthest-reaching searches in history have been expeditions to the depths of the ocean, missions in the outer limits of space and, most awe-inspiring of all, the hunt for the perfect lipstick.

Go on, laugh. But in all my years of dealing with the public, that's been the question that's gotten asked the most (well, next to, "Can you make me look 20 years younger in the next 10 minutes?"). Everybody seems to wind up with a shade that's either too light or too dark, too hot or too cool, too sheer or too opaque, too this, too that or too something else entirely. "Just right," it seems, is the Holy Grail of lipstick.

Mind you, I'm not making fun here. I'm only trying to make *you* have fun. I know that lipstick is serious business. But it doesn't have to be *that* serious. It's an impulse, not a human pulse, so relax; it's not sink-or-swim (contrary to the way it may feel, there's a lot of perfectly acceptable dog-paddling that can be done). And the sooner you realize that you'll never find the right shade (that is, the shade that you will like next week, next season or next year as much as you

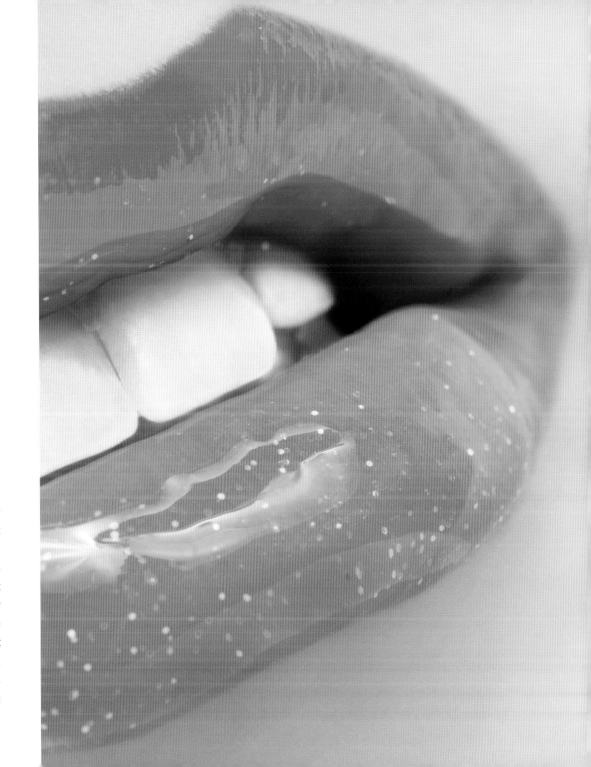

did yesterday), the happier you will be. And the more likely you will be to start (that's right) having fun with the never-ending search.

Ultimately, lipstick is dictated almost as much by your mood as it is by your color preference, its texture and hue suggestive of your frame of mind in the instant that you purchased the tube. Did you need a pick-me-up? Were you feeling va-va-va-voomy … or did you want to feel that way later? Your lips will tell the tale without your ever having to move them. (For some of us, I know, making a decision is like getting a root canal, only without the laughing gas to keep the anxiety at bay. But think of it this way: After conquering brows, lipstick is going to come as naturally to you as smooching.)

You should also bear in mind that lipstick comes in more formulas than you're likely to find on a mad scientist's drawing board. This is not meant to torture you (and certainly not in the same way that eyebrow plucking is). That's just technology … progress … fun! The sooner you surrender to the fact that your high-school sweetheart's waistline is likelier to remain the same than lipstick formulas, the sooner you will be able to enjoy the wild ride on which their conjurers intend to take us. That said, I prefer a simple cream formula and a summer sheer with an SPF 15; it's easy and far from a lifetime commitment.

(So much for advances in science, huh?)

As for application … well, you're going to like this part. If selecting your lipstick gets you all wound up, then at least applying it will help you wind back down. Step one involves your old friend, the mirror. Look into it with your mouth closed and relaxed (no lip-pursing, no matter how much the decision-making process gave you agita). Next, take a coordinating matching pencil and lipstick, and, starting at the corner of the mouth, slowly draw a line up to the middle. Then, softly round out the peak of the lip (or the cupid's bow). Then, do the same thing on the other side (unless your intention is to exact a sort of Dr. Jekyll and Ms. Hyde look), meeting in the middle.

Now, smile ever so slightly, and color your lower lip simply by following its natural line. The job of your liner is to shape, define and, maybe most importantly, give you a guide to follow while filling in the color that you have chosen. (In a way, it turns your mouth into a coloring book; all you have to do is stay within the lines!) After filling in your color, step back and take a close look at your handiwork: Make sure you have the lipstick evenly distributed. If so, you're good (maybe even great) to go. If not, take a Q-Tip and balance yourself out first.

If your mouth is too small or you have no upper lip to speak of, just lean the pencil on the outside edge of your natural lip line; the result will amaze you. And if your lips are too large for your liking, or your lower one appears to have been supersized, try leaning the pencil to the inside of the natural lip line. Also, remember that the color you choose can make a small lip look bigger or a big lip look bigger still (and vice-versa). So, if you are trying to remedy something that you consider to be a flaw, it's best to go with a softer shade, thereby drawing less attention to your area of concern.

Finally, a couple of helpful hints. First off, I sometimes use gloss to make a lower lip pop; all you have to do is put it in the center of your lower lip. This next trick was taught to me by none other than *As the World Turns'* knockout Colleen Zenk Pinter: Take a white pencil and run it along the top lip softly, blending so as to bring a highlight (and thus, everybody's attention) to the area. (It really works, but then, if you've ever so much as seen a picture of Colleen, you already know that!) Of course, you could probably live without these little tricks, but why would you want to? Trust me, these tricks are treats!

As we seal this chapter with the proverbial kiss, I'd like to add one last reminder: This make-up stuff doesn't all fall into place at once. Nope. Like you yourself, your face is a work in progress, so don't bother freaking out if you aren't a master of the game overnight. This game is just too darn unwieldy … like Life. Luckily, it's not a matter of Life … and death.

EVA TAMARGO

I've got to be honest with you, folks. When I met Eva Tamargo, I didn't like her. Nope. I *loved* her. Seriously, she has this energy about her that draws you to her like a magnet. Even if the Brooklyn native wasn't a self-professed shoe-whore (which she is—which, of course, made her catnip to me), I still would've followed her around like a besotted puppy. She's got her you-know-what together, and the effect is, in a word, hot. So I wasn't surprised in the least to discover that, in the mid-1990s, telenovelas tripped over one another fighting to be the next Spanish-language soap to cast her as a femme fatale. What *did* surprise me was finding out just how dowdy her *Passions* character is: Not only did poor Pilar Lopez-Fitzgerald spend years cleaning up after the filthy rich, but her kids are, like, old! (One of her former on-screen offspring is muscle-bound Jesse Metcalfe, aka *Desperate Housewives'* resident bush-wacker). Beyond the suds, the onetime acting student of *Law & Order's* Sam Waterston has done films (including the box-office touch-down *Any Given Sunday*), primetime and even reality TV (as host of a *casa*-improvement show). Through it all, though, it seems she's learned her most important lessons are not about her craft but about life. Keep reading, and you'll see what I mean.

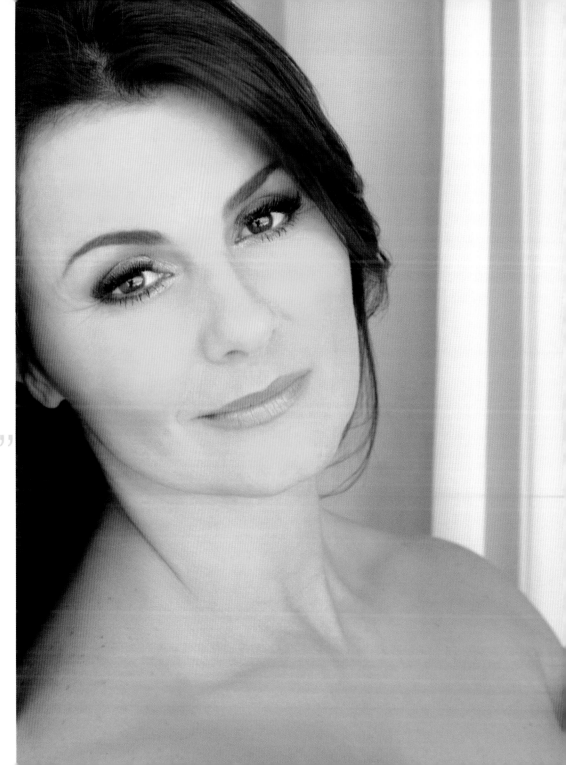

"I AM
COMMITTED
TO MY
CONVICTIONS"

EVA TAMARGO

Please tell me that while your *Passions* character's husband was "dead," they let her have a little love life.
No. Never. I'm very loyal. I guess that's one of the more admirable parts to my character. She truly believed in her heart that even if he's not there, you still remain loyal.

Not even one flirtation?
No. Now, *children*, on the other hand … *(Laughs)* They want Pilar to have a few!

How old are your TV kids?
My gosh, they range from early 30s to 20s.

(Looks hard at Eva) Nope. I just don't get that.
Me neither! But my character is very conservative. I don't look like this on the show, ever!

I can't believe they don't take advantage of how glamorous you are. I mean, I can tell—in real life, you're a sexpot! Totally over-the-top!
Oh, yes, yes. It is kind of funny that they put me in this role. When I first read for it, I knew it was a mom role, but I thought I would be the mother of a 9-year-old. So when I saw my "kids," I said, "Whaaat?" It's interesting how things happen, though. At first, I thought this was so not me, but that's when I was comparing Pilar to the superficial side [of myself]. I actually have a lot of similar qualities to Pilar. I'm very loyal, very maternal and very committed to my convictions. I don't sway.

Putting aside Pilar for a moment, what does beauty mean to you?
I've come into this as I've gotten older—it's finally accepting yourself. That is beauty. That's the most beautiful thing you can see in a woman, because you can see someone who's actually drop-dead gorgeous who has no self-esteem, no self-assurance, no confidence, no voice. So I feel more beautiful today, and I don't mean superficially, because I've learned to own all my crap and my baggage.

That which doesn't kill us makes us not only stronger but prettier, too.
Yeah, that is beautiful when you see someone and go, "Wow, look at the way she carries herself!"

Exactly. On the flip side, I hate it when I'm watching an award show and see a woman whose dress is wearing her instead of the other way around.
I totally agree. But in their defense, [that self-awareness is] something that comes later in life. I mean, when I was in my 20s, I was very angry. But if you're smart and you're learning from all these experiences, you come to this. I heard Oprah Winfrey say recently, because she'd just turned 50, "I thought I had my s—-together in my 40s. *Now* I have it together. And 10 years from now, I'll say, 'Oh, wait a minute.'" Every decade, every phase of your life, has enchantments and disappointments.

Sometimes those lessons are hard to learn.
Hard. But sometimes tough love is needed, man.

What's the hardest lesson you've ever learned?
To be honest, I think it would be that fantasy that we all buy into about your [knight in] shining armor and that love lasts forever … that *everything* lasts forever. You know, we're on borrowed time. I'm getting divorced, and my husband and I are very amicable, but knocking yourself off that …

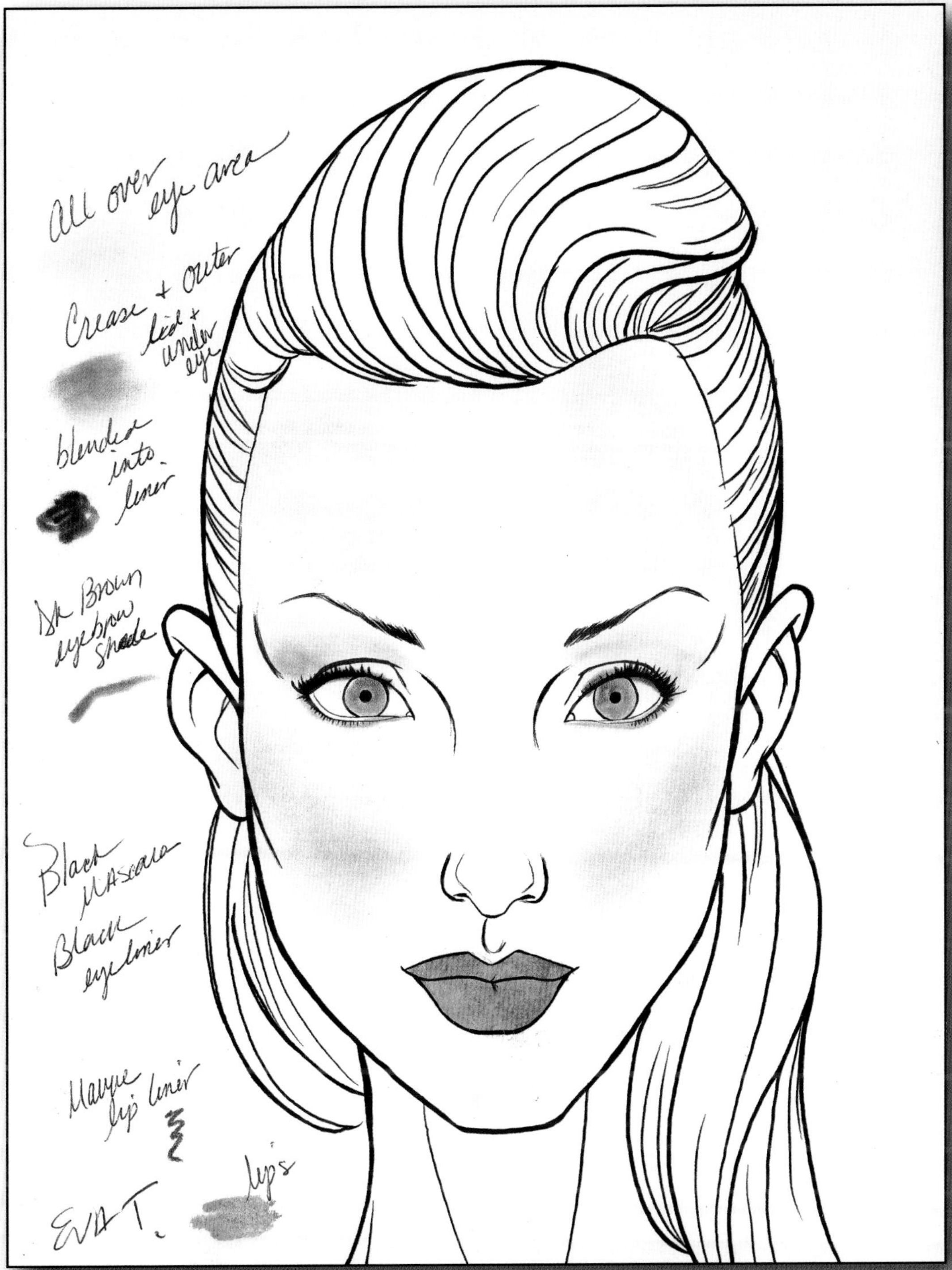

All over eye area

Crease + Outer lid + under eye

blended into liner

Dk Brown eyebrow shade

Black MAscara

Black eyeliner

Mauve lip liner

EVA T. lips

That illusion of happily ever after?

It's not that you go into a marriage and say, "Well, this might end in divorce," but there's a certain idealistic quality that women tend to lean toward that it's always going to be beautiful and perfect. That's the biggest lesson I've learned. Not that life is difficult, but it's full of ups and downs.

Is there anything missing from the world today that you wish we could get back?

To be honest with you, because my parents are older, what comes up for me is respect. There is no respect, in every aspect—in the workplace, in the family, children to parents, respect for the elderly. I just read a thing about getting older in our society, and that it's your fault, but hello?! What about all the great things about getting old? You're *supposed* to get older.

If I'm not, I'm doing something very wrong! (Laughs) Riddle me this: If I were to open your make-up box, what would I find? All neutrals? All glamour? Or a little bit of everything?

My make-up is very neutral. I'm not a big make-up person. The only "must" things in my make-up bag are my eyelash curler and mascara.

You do have gorgeous eyes.

Oh, thank you. Now that I'm a little bit older, I do wear a little bit of tinted foundation and a sunblock. But I'm really pretty down-to-earth. It's indicative of my whole personality. I'm very much jeans and boots; I'm an artisan. But I love make-up, too. Like today [at this shoot], I love getting made up and all that.

You're my dream model, because what I want women to walk away from this book with is the fact that they can have everything. Be down-to-earth, yes, but be able to pull out all the stops whenever you want to.

Make-up to me really doesn't always say who you really are. It enhances parts of you, but some women can't see beyond that. They can't see themselves outside of their make-up. [They think] people won't accept them, because they can't accept themselves without make-up.

They're hiding. Which is okay every now and again.

As long as you're hiding in a fun way. It's all about balance.

Anything you'd like to add?

I just want to leave people, especially women, with something that I found somewhere, and I have it on my wall. "And the older I get, the older I've gotten, the more I feel like myself."

Very nice.

I look in the mirror sometimes, and I go, "Where is that little girl in her 20s? She was so scared." We look at youth [without realizing that] only the physical part is what you want. I don't want to be in that physical plane, you know what I mean? The older I get, the more this is the Eva I've always wanted to be. It's not an act anymore. That's my energy. I don't have anything to hide.

KATHERINE KELLY LANG

When I met Katherine Kelly Lang for our photo shoot, it was late at night, she'd been working since God knows when, and, immediately after we were done, she was heading off to God knows where. Okay, I know where—Italy. The point is, she should have been *nuts*. But she wasn't, and as a result, I was utterly fascinated. Warm, calm and collected, she sat down with me for an intimate conversation that, had time permitted, I suspect would have gone on for hours. And making up her face? Let me put it this way: Even if it hadn't been after dark, I might have thought I was dreaming. Simply put, she epitomizes the titular concept of *The Bold & the Beautiful,* where, since the soap's 1987 debut, she has played the frequently harried and *more* frequently married Brooke Logan. (To include all of her character's last names would require a chapter unto itself.) Even before coming to daytime, she seemed destined for stardom. The daughter of actors Judith Lang and Keith Wegeman—that's the Jolly Green Giant to you and me—the native Californian turned up as a youngster on classic series like *Happy Days* and *Magnum, P.I.* Then, after a short stint as Gretchen on *The Young & the Restless,* sister soap *B&B* made her its waitress-turned-chemist-turned-Lady Trump. None of which explains where she gets her sense of serenity, however. Perhaps if you read between the lines of our chat, you'll form your own opinion. Me? Oh, you know me—I was having too good a time for analysis.

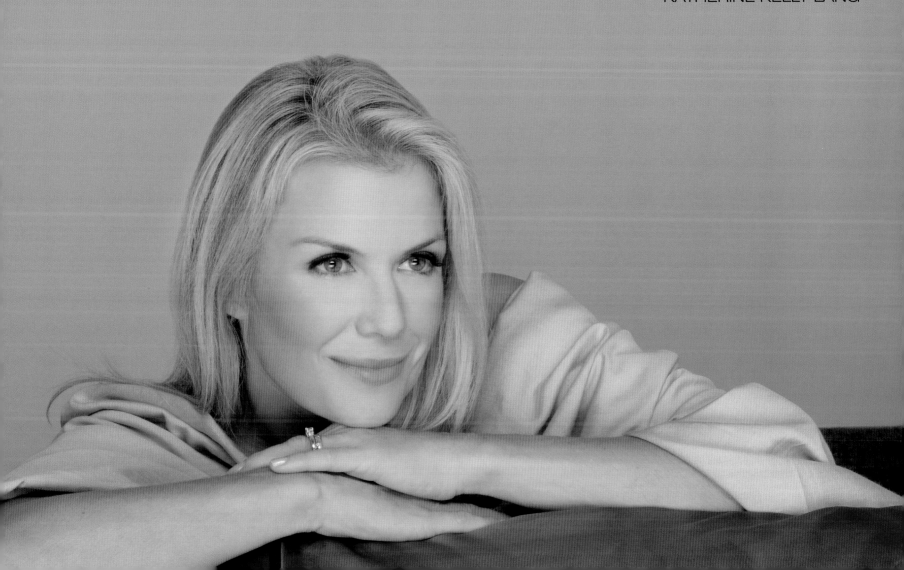

"IT'S TAKEN ME YEARS TO LEARN HOW TO DO EYELINER"

KATHERINE KELLY LANG

What does beauty mean to you?

Beauty, to me, comes from the inside. If you're gorgeous but not happy on the inside, you don't feel good about yourself, and that's going to show. A lot of it comes from your perspective on life. Also, what you eat and drink. Then, of course, there's outside beauty, which is different for everybody. Different styles, different looks …

True. In some cultures, I am considered prettier than Ryan Phillippe. Do you believe that make-up has power?

Yes, it accentuates all the right places. The eyes, especially, and the lips and of course the cheekbones. It does help.

At what age did you realize the power of a woman?

That's a good question. I'm trying to think of moments with my dad, but I'm not sure the "woman thing" came in with that. If you want to say "woman," it's definitely more in my late teens.

Let's talk about *The Bold & the Beautiful* a bit. Who was Brooke's best husband?

(Laughs) Fantasy-wise?

Character-wise.

I would say Ridge (played by Ronn Moss).

And you've been with him for what … 12 years now?

Well, we weren't married for a couple of years, and I've been married to him a couple times. But we finally have a child together. So this would be the most successful marriage as of now. I mean, it could be terrible tomorrow!

You could just as easily be talking about clothes as marriages. I was surfing the Web for some old photos of you, and apparently, Brooke used to be really into suits with linebacker shoulder pads.

She had the business look going for a while.

Which she alternated with a vast array of barely-there negligees.

[She went between] the Armani look and Brooke's Bedroom [outfits], which meant parading around in her [own line of] lingerie.

What was your favorite look?

Well, the lingerie scenes are always a little stressful, but she also has some very sexy, glamorous gowns and dresses which I like.

Have you ever had to redo a scene because your lipstick smeared?

I'm sure that has happened, but I don't want to say it was just my lipstick in particular; it could have been any part of my make-up. Also my hair. That used to be a big one with one of our producers. She'd see one hair out of place, and we would have to stop right in the middle of a scene.

Who gives better catfight—Hunter Tylo (who played Taylor Forrester, Brooke's virtuous rival for Ridge's affections) or Susan Flannery (who plays her monster-in-law, Stephanie)?

Susan Flannery, definitely. *(Laughs)*

Who's your favorite leading man?

I'd have to say Ronn. I've worked with him more since day one than anybody. We always gel in a good way. And he's always easy and comforting to work with. He has a very positive, relaxing personality. Very supportive.

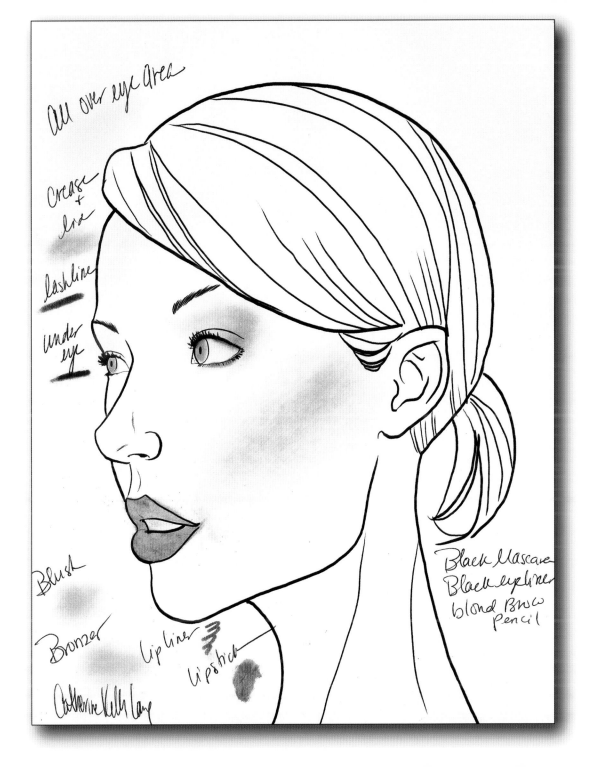

All over eye area

Crease + lid

lashline

under eye

Blush

Bronzer

Catherine Kelly Lang

Lipliner

Lipstick

Black Mascara
Black eyeliner
blond Brow
pencil

Aside from going nine rounds in character with Susan Flannery, do you have a favorite guilty pleasure?

Chocolate.

And a favorite late-night treat—or did you just answer that question, too?

My pillow.

What are you most proud of?

My kids.

You have four, right?

Yes, three of my own and my stepdaughter.

How old is your stepdaughter?

She's 13. My two sons are 14 and 11, and my other daughter is 7.

They must keep you hopping! Do you ever, I dunno, pick up a make-up book to kick back and relax?

No.

But you'll read this one, won't you?

Honestly?

Unless your answer is going to be no.

Yes, I will. I just have never been able to do my make-up too well. It's taken me years to learn just how to do decent eyeliner and mascara.

This should be an interesting question then—who influenced you the most where beauty is concerned?

My mother. She had a very organic hippie kind of flair, which is where I got my style, from her. But when it comes to high fashion, I definitely got that from magazines.

So, would you say that you're the ultimate California girl?

Yes, wearing my jeans and my T-shirt, no make-up, my hair pulled back in a ponytail …

Considering how much time you had to have spent on the beach, you've got gorgeous skin. How have you managed to protect it so well?

I kind of abused my skin by being in the sun my whole life. Many days, I never put on sunscreen. But I've been trying to take better care of it. I get facials, and I'm trying to find the right creams for my face, things like that. I think that eating healthy, drinking a lot of water, and taking certain vitamins help the skin, too.

If that's what you've been doing, I have to say I wholeheartedly agree.

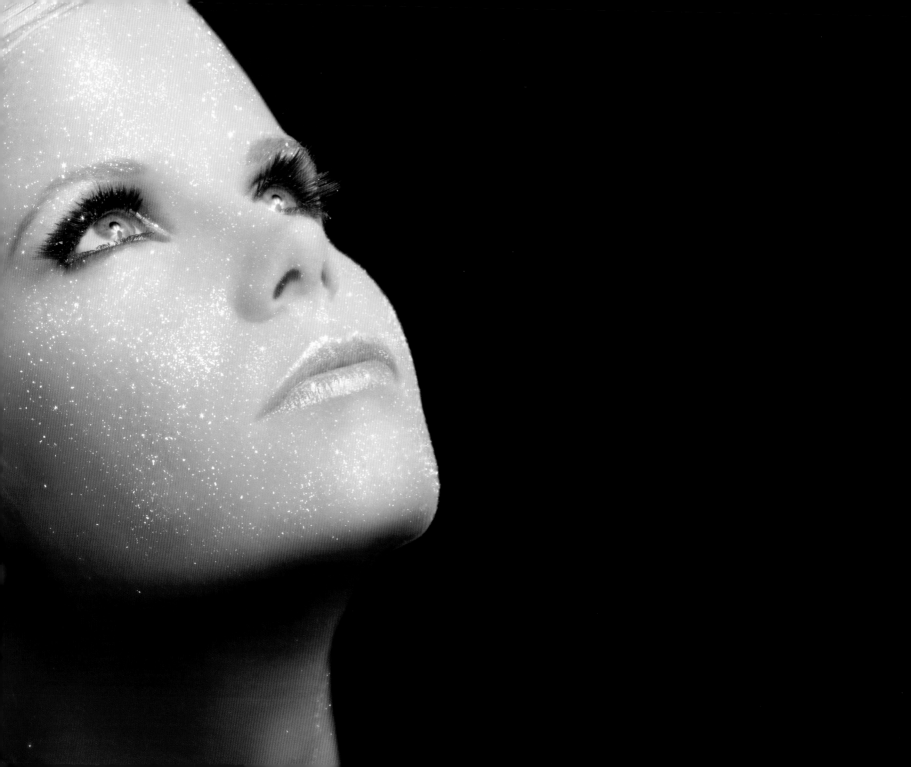

CHAPTER 8:

Night and Day

If you were a soap character, you might put on a wig, boa and a phony accent to distinguish your everyday self from your night-on-the-town self. But since you're not we are going to take a simpler approach that is no less dazzling.

Would I Lie to You

Before we dive in, though, you will need one thing: a good grasp on your everyday face. No, this does not mean to take your head in your hands the way we have done in other chapters. This means you have to take a good look at yourself. See? That's not so hard, is it? After that, the rest is gravy … or groovy. Or … oh, you know what I mean. It's going to be no-brainer stuff, and it's going to look awesome!

Now then, if you've seen all the fun beauty products lining the shelves—and who are we kidding? I know you have!—you know that you can really cut loose—or you can rein yourself in, picking and choosing only the items you care to try. One rule, though: No more Tammy Faye Baker lashes! Her comfort level with her outer look was very cool, but she's her own artist and owes no more explanation for her cosmetic exploits than does Picasso for his adventures on canvas. By contrast, you can also do very, very little in the way of make-up and still have glamour out the wazoo. Just look at *One Life to Live's* young Kristen Alderson: That kid has style to spare, but at her age, she's not ready for a fraction of the glosses and add-ons other can consider.

SPEAKING OF WHICH, AMONG THE COOLER COSMETICS THAT YOU MIGHT WANT TO SAMPLE ARE:

Glitter liners with bases that you can use to line your top lashes. They can add a subtle glimmer or an overwhelming sparkle, depending on the shade you use and (Lord knows) how much of it you use. (I imagine it's the difference between the showgirl look and the intergalactic party-girl look.)

Shimmer liquids that you can pour into your foundation (in moderation, of course), resulting in, you know, that glow. After all, what's the point in waiting till you've arrived in the hereafter to radiate a celestial warmth? By then, everybody will have it!

False eyelashes. I know, I know: I just got done saying that the Tammy Faye look is reserved exclusively for Tammy Faye. But there is a happy medium. I love false eyelashes—and not just on RuPaul, either. Despite their reputation as being a preferred accessory of streetwalkers and mannequins, they can make you look truly special for a special occasion. Or, for you math majors reading this, it's like your regular ol' eyes times 10—but with less make-up!

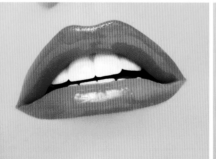
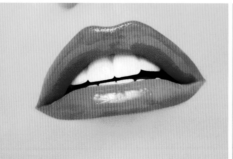
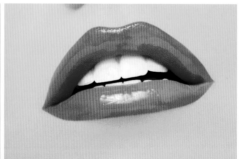
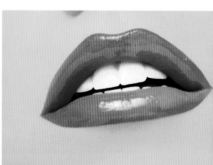

You can kill a whole afternoon simply by stopping by a department-store make-up counter and asking the resident expert to see their wildest new looks for evening. In no time, the two of you will be having a blast. (If you're not, try another counter; you may have wandered into a morgue.) Just remember: Even if you are in charge nowhere else in your life, at the counter you're the boss! No clerk can tell you that you must make a purchase. Or rather, they can tell you that, I suppose, but it's not true; in fact, usually, it's against store policy. Why? Because make-up is supposed to be fun, and if you are having fun with make-up, you will want to buy some.

Are we having fun, or what? (Please don't answer "or what," because we're turning the last corner here, and if you aren't having fun yet, you probably aren't going to, and that, neither I nor my therapist are equipped to handle.)

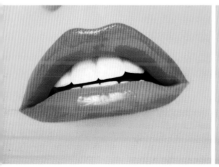 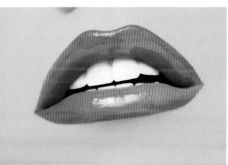 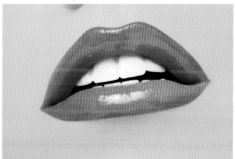 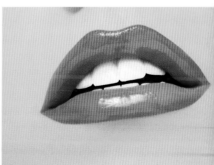

AMELIA MARSHALL

When I look at Amelia Marshall, I see classical elegance—the lady was made for descending magnificent staircases in the kind of ballgowns that are only designed by fairy godmothers. But, having worked with her for years, I know that the qualities that make her so easy on the eyes can't hold a candle to the ones she possesses that make her so delightful to the heart. Don't get me wrong—she *is* elegant. (Bette Davis, forgive me, but the silver-screen sirens of Hollywood's Golden Age have nothin' on this Broadway scene-stealer.) However, she is also modest and unassuming, as pure a soul as you are likely to encounter this far down to Earth. In her first soap roles, as plucky good girls Gilly Grant on *Guiding Light* and Belinda Keefer on *All My Children*, she proudly let her innate sweetness come out. Yet it is only since she doffed the Ms. Nice Guy sash to play *Passions*' vindictive Liz Sanbourne that she's knocked daytime fans off the edge of their seats and onto the floor. The funny thing is, it doesn't seem to be only viewers who are getting a kick out of her character's antics—she is, too! Talking recently with the single mom, she seemed, even more so than usual, utterly at home in her supple skin. Keep reading, and you'll soon know what I mean.

"BEAUTY COMES FROM YOUR HEART"

AMELIA MARSHALL

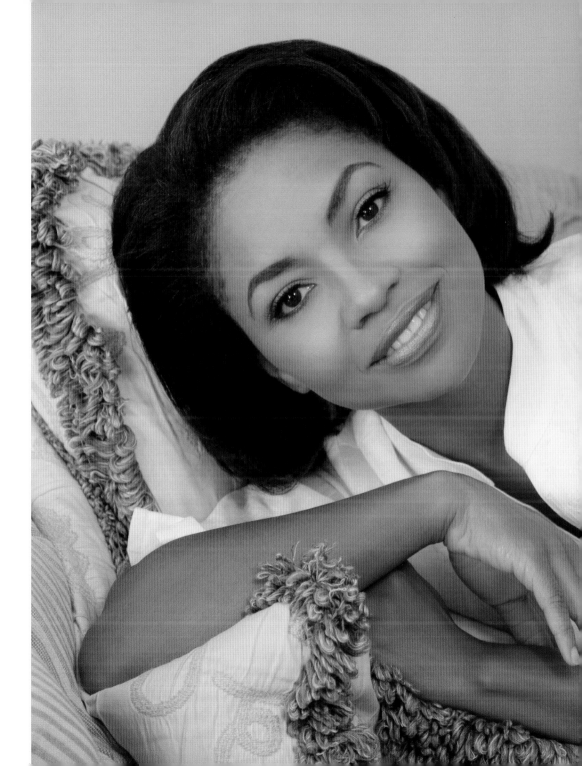

On a scale of fat-free brownies to cheesecake, how much fun are you having playing *Passions'* Liz?
She's such a bitch! *(Laughs)* She is! I've never played a character like this before. And ...

And you're *so* not like that!
… which allows you to explore that and just let it go. There have been times when I've drawn the line, but I just try to have fun with that.

I think that's really reflected in your new look, too; it's far less buttoned-down than your other characters.
Yeah, you don't worry about the hair or the beauty aspect as much. I can just go in to get my revenge.
Plus, her hair has a slightly less tamed look, which feeds into the character.

How cool for you to be able to reinvent yourself this way! Of course, whenever I've seen you, no matter who you've been playing, you've always turned heads. Where does your sense of beauty come from? Wherever it is, other people should frequent that place!
It comes from your heart [and], to me, from feeling a part of the world but not of the world. There's this thing about seeing the smile on a child's face and knowing that you had something to do with that. It's superficial … transient.

Unless it comes from the inside out, in which case …
… it comes not so much from confidence about your looks but more out of the confidence that I'm doing the best I can every day, for me, for my family, for my fellow man.

Can you imagine if everybody lived that way?
That would be really cool.

So, aside from putting one foot—your best foot—forward and in front of the other, beauty-wise, how do you prepare to go out into the world?
I'm not one to put on make-up before I go out. You'll see me in Target with hopefully some moisturizer on, but that's about it. *(Laughs)*

Who taught you the most about beauty in your life?
Interesting. I don't think it was my mom or my grandmother, who I can't even remember wearing make-up. It was never really about that. As far as my mom was concerned, if your body was clean and your clothes were pressed and your hair was neatly combed, you were presentable. So it has always been sort of basics for me. I remember when I first moved to New York, I was feeling very much the insecurity that comes with moving to a huge city and suddenly being bombarded with auditions, which are a real and intense sort of judgment situation.

How did you handle it?
Well, my roommate at the time was this beautiful, shapely young woman who men just dropped dead over. I remember going to a party with another girlfriend and my roommate, and when we walked in, all the men stared at her. I told my girlfriend, "You know, sometimes I feel so unattractive," and she goes, "What are you talking about? Your beauty is in you—it's not about boobs! It's in you, and it comes out." No one had ever told me that.

That's an especially nice story to hear since women so often seem to tear each other down rather than build each other up.
It was such a gift. Now I really look beyond the package: If you're content with who you are from the inside, you're going to be just fine. I can remember after a divorce going, "Oooh! Oooh!"

Ouch. That's gotta turn your world around on its axis.
It does. It pulls the rug out from underneath you. Whatever you predicted for the future is no longer there. You have to

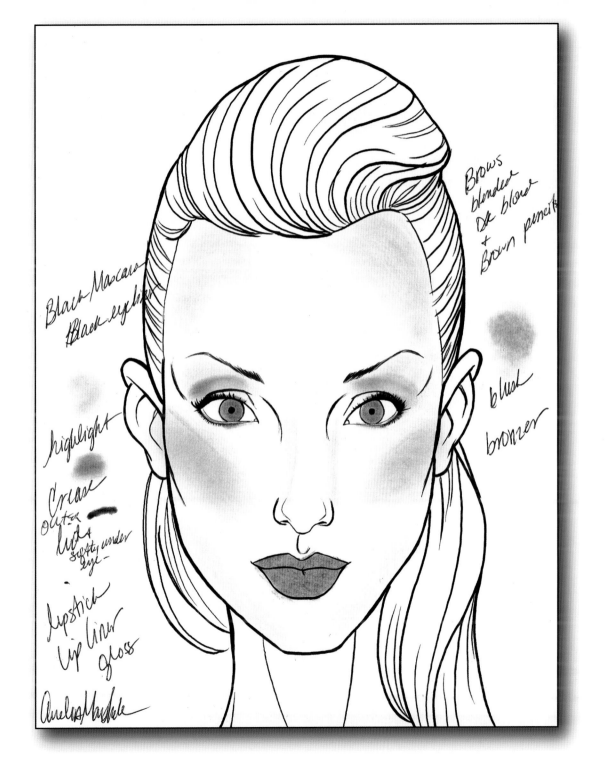

Brows blended Dk blond + Brown pencils

Black Mascara + Black eyeliner

blush

bronzer

highlight

Crease
Outer Lids softly under eye

Lipstick
Lip liner
gloss

one
hundred
thirty**one**

rebuild. I remember going back to dance, refinding my passions that had been the driving force of my life, and suddenly having that happiness come in. Again, you start to feel beautiful, and it doesn't really matter what the exterior is.

I wish young girls got that message louder and clearer earlier on, before they start prematurely experimenting with make-up.
When you're young, you don't even need make-up. You've got everything pumping—you've got this glorious skin, and if you're eating right and drinking all this water, you've got all this color in your face. It's weird to me to see painted girls at the amusement park, at the mall, at the beach …

At the gym!
I mean, where are you going? That's so L.A. I'm not sure why our society has done this. Why would MTV and all these shows lay this on young girls? I remember trying out for Broadway shows [right after I got to Manhattan], and a friend pulled me over and said, "Just go to a department store—they'll teach you how to put base on." And I did! *(Laughs)*

And did they?
Yeah! When I moved to New York, I still looked like I was 14, because of good genes. [Casting people] actually thought I was younger than I was, so I needed to put on make-up to look older. But if you're 14, you don't need to look older! If you're really 14, be 14!

Did you have trouble finding base when you first started wearing it? Or were you mixing it yourself back then?
I did, but there were two companies, Florie Roberts and Fashion Fair. I was between those two colors, and depending on whether it was summer or winter, you mixed it accordingly. Every black woman I knew did that.

I still have Fashion Fair and Florie Roberts in my bag—they're staples.
Sure, and even now, there is a company that will do a custom blend by computer.

In the past, I've actually called companies and asked them what are darker skin-toned girls supposed to do for base? But they didn't care. They said that they base everything on a national sales level, and since darker-complected girls don't necessarily wear base, they don't bother to make it. Thank God things are changing.
It's difficult. It's going to take a little while longer to mix your base in the morning rather than just pop a bottle open and put it on, then you're out the door. I'm always fascinated by the Iman line because it's so olive-toned. It's hard for me to wear, because anything with an olive tint, I'm in trouble.

You ash?
Yup, and it looks like I'm ill. It takes away all the color from my skin. I'm yellow-red, and I need that to look healthy.

Let's get serious again for a moment. What do you think is missing in the world today that we once had?
Innocence. As you grow older, you are aware of how much we're bombarded with. Certainly, 9/11 was having the innocence and arrogance of America being ripped away. Personally, in the last three years, because I've had family members close to death, I've lost some of that irrational innocence of saying that I know this loved one is going to live forever; you have to come to terms with the fact that they're not. It's interesting when you have a young child, and you see their innocence …

It's bittersweet, isn't it? Because you know what lies ahead.
Yeah. You just want to say, "Enjoy it, enjoy it, enjoy it!"

And don't be so quick to grow up!
Which gets you back to those girls who just want to be older. Don't be so in a hurry! Enjoy where you are!

PATRIKA DARBO

When I first got the idea to write this book, I immediately thought of my soap-star friends to be in it. But I also thought of someone else … someone I'd never actually met: Patrika Darbo. Maybe it's because she *seemed* like somebody I'd be friends with. She certainly seemed like someone everybody has in their lives—and I don't mean to imply that she's common, either. What I'm getting at is the fact that, unlike so many of the women I (and, no doubt, you) see on TV, she seems less a figment of a writer or plastic surgeon's imagination and more … well, real. Vivacious and warm and real. And to my astonishment, despite my high expectations, she didn't disappoint. She was as down-to-earth as an angel can be. And, while I was excited to have her as a part of this project because she's made such an impact as *Days of Our Lives*' reformed pot-stirrer, Nancy Wesley, her list of accomplishments goes way beyond the soaps. Gee, where to begin? She recurred on the classic sitcom *Growing Pains* and was a regular on *Step by Step*, with Patrick Duffy and Suzanne Somers; she's guest-starred on everything from *Seinfeld* to *Roseanne*, and even *played* the former Mrs. Tom Arnold in the tell-all bio *Roseanne & Tom: Behind the Scenes*; and her film credits include the sequel to *Speed*, *Daddy's Dyin' … Who's Got the Will?* and *Mr. and Mrs. Smith*, with Brad Pitt and Angelina Jolie. And here's my favorite of her credits: She voiced one of the sheep in the original *Babe*. (All together now: Awwww!) An avid writer, she is also the author of the titillatingly titled, ultimately empowering self-help book, *365 Glorious Nights of Love and Romance*. Can you tell I felt very lucky to spend one glorious afternoon of love and cosmetics with her? Read on, and believe me when I say that you're gonna fall for her, too.

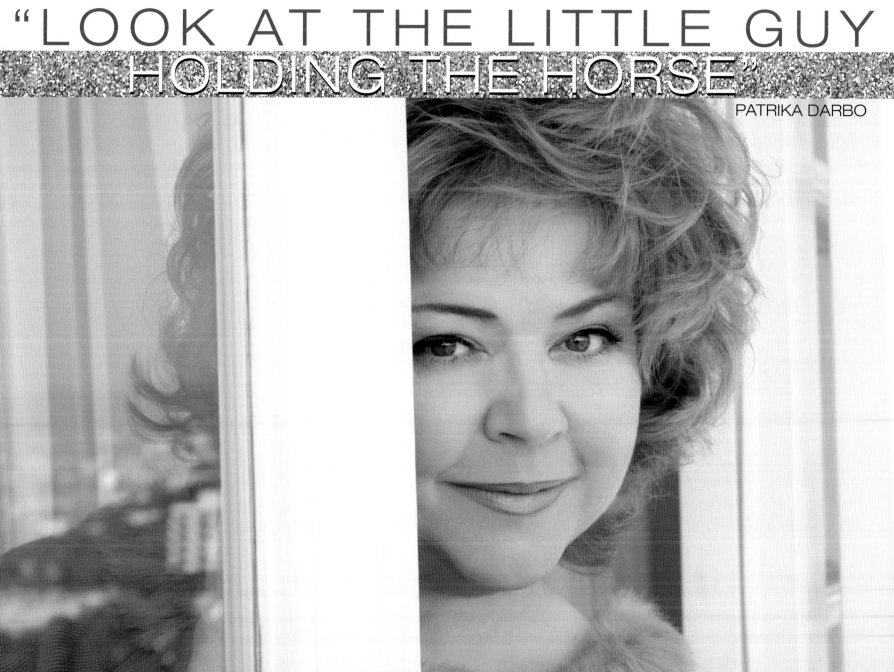

"LOOK AT THE LITTLE GUY HOLDING THE HORSE"

PATRIKA DARBO

**I remember reading about you once in _TV Guide_. I think the term they used to describe Nancy was "bitch goddess."
Were you sorry when she mellowed?**

Well, getting to be mean was very nice. I've always played the beat-up housewife, so this was the first time that I not only got to play the bad woman but also the sexual woman, which was …

Every woman's fantasy.

It is, but it's in all of us. I think what happens is we fall victim to what we see on television as far as the ads telling us that we are less than perfect if we have 10 extra pounds or if we have a bit of acne. I was very fortunate that my dad said you can be anything you want to be. And my dad was only 4'2". He was known as the biggest little man in baseball. I had that kind of going for me.

Was your dad a baseball player?

He was in the front office, with the Boston Braves/Milwaukee Braves/Atlanta Braves. Not that it was the coolest childhood, but still, I had the good things in it. People would call it a dysfunctional family, but we all come from dysfunctional families in one way or another.

If we were all perfect, we'd never learn anything.

I mean, I think I am who I am because of [my upbringing]. And I think I'm a good person, a nice person.

So far, I would have to agree. _(Laughs)_ But back to Nancy for a moment …

It was like, "Why live vicariously through a size 2 when you can now live vicariously through a size 20?" And now you don't have to live vicariously at all, because I _am_ you. The best part about it is that [on the show], I had this fabulous, fantastically soap-opera good-looking husband who worshipped the ground I walked on. And never was weight an issue. He was knocking me down, doing me in the parking lot. I was knocking him down, doing him in the parking lot, in the closet, in the hospital, in the hot tub … everywhere. We were not only a nonstereotypical couple, but we had everything that a very typical couple does have.

And until Kathy Brier came along on _One Life to Live_, you were the only one who had done it.

I'm very happy to be doing that. Nobody ever had a problem with John Goodman being married to a size 2, so why is that acceptable and [a heavier wife] isn't?

Hell if I know! Is that one of the things you address in your book?

Well, my book is basically about how I got started in the business, and that this is the package I come in, so put a bow on and get out there. Don't sit at home wasting your life, because life flies by much too fast. I also tell women that basically, everyone is looking for the white knight. Take a look at the little guy holding the horse because he may be worshipping the ground you walk on, and you're not even looking at him.

That is so sweet.

That's a very important thing. We all want someone, but from the same medium that's telling us that we're not perfect, we're being told to look for the white knight.

It's senseless! Let's hit some beauty questions. What does the word mean to you?

Beauty means to me a friendly, nice person. They could have the worst acne in the world, they could have a scar across their face, they could have no arms and one leg, but if they have a warm smile … well, I think beauty means a smile. And eyes that say, "Hello, how are you? Glad to meet you." Not somebody who looks at you and simply goes dead.

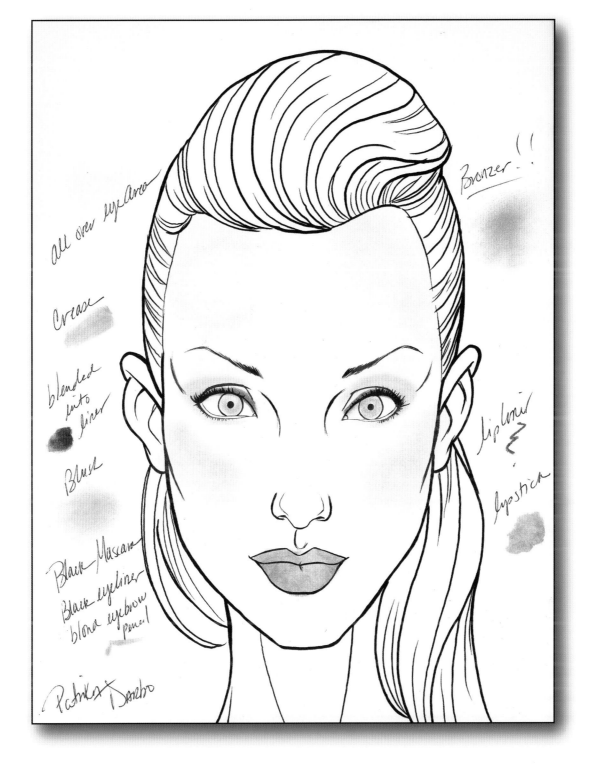

Who taught you the most about beauty?

My [late] mother [although] she was my worst enemy at the same time. She took my head shot across the room once and told someone that she was prettier than me. So I come from that kind of thing. I think my husband [has taught me a lot about beauty, too]. We've been married for 31 years, and he loves me thin, fat, bad-hair day, good-hair day, chicken pox, flu, a bitch day, whatever. He can look past anything and still give me that warm, fuzzy feeling … that hug. I could just come to him and say I need attention, and I would get it. But I think at that first Weight Watchers meeting that I ever went to, Virginia Lamb … She was the first one who said that you are worthwhile whether this [diet] succeeds or not.

I'm glad you were able to really hear her. Do you believe that make-up has power?

Oh, absolutely, because I think there are times when you really feel like doo-doo, and just adding lipstick releases something in your whole being that gives you something. It's interesting, because sometimes, when I think you're feeling your worst you do your best make-up job.

I'm envious of women, because they have that luxury.

If I just add lipstick, I feel like I can go anywhere and do anything, because I look good. And then a hint of mascara, and you own the world. If any woman's pocketbook has lipstick and mascara in it, she can own the world.

What is the hardest lesson you've every learned?

That I can't be perfect and that I am my own worst enemy for trying to be. I think that that's something that everyone needs to learn. It's like finding out that somebody doesn't like you. That's devastating. But somebody said to me one time, "Do you *like* everybody? No? Then why do you expect everybody to like you?" You can't spend your energy on someone who's not worth it. That's the hardest lesson. I'm not sure I'm there yet, but I'm working toward it.

What's been your favorite storyline on the show?

Working with Lisa Linde (*X-Men* hottie James Marsden's wife, who played off-kilter Ali) and Kevin Spirtas (who played Nancy's doctor spouse, Mike), when we were trying to drive her nuts and have my husband become chief-of-staff. We were in bed together, we were in trash barrels together, we were running across the States … We had a good time.

Is Kevin your favorite leading man?

It's between him and Beau Bridges. Beau Bridges, I'd lay down in front of a train for; I think he's wonderful. But Kevin has been one of those people who has made me turn down the tape player of all the old tapes and create new ones. He's made me go sing with him, he's made me dress up. He's just a very good friend. I adore him.

Any classic embarrassing moments on the show?

My most embarrassing moment was having to go to the guy who was filling up the hot tub and say, "Now, you know I'm going to displace more water than if Kristian Alfonso (who plays svelte Hope) got in it." I was mortified. I was thinking I was going to get in this hot tub, and the water was going to spill out the side. I also told the [crew] when I found out we had to jump through a window to measure my butt, because I didn't want any problems when I had to go through.

Is there anything missing from the world today that you wish you could get back?

My parents. There are unsaid things that will never be said now.

What is your biggest waste of time?

Television. I'm a junkie. If I can't see it, then I tape it and watch it later. I can tell people what shows are going to make it or not make it. I'm a good judge of that. I'm sorry to say that I love to watch Emeril cook, but I was so offended by the ads when the heavyweight black girl was chewing on chocolate cake and then wanted more cake. I will not do a stereotypical fat joke. If someone's sitting at home in Iowa not laughing, it's not funny. It may be funny to all you thin people, but I'm not doing it. Thank you very much, good-bye, I'm outta here. And I let my agents know that.

Good for you. You're recurring at *Days* now. Anything else in the pipeline?

I'm writing and hope to produce some things coming up. I have this show called *Green Pastures*, which, in short, is about a young woman whose brother and sister-in-law are killed on the eve of her being ordained as a minister, and so she gets their kids. She's now a mother, and she's moving to a new town to get her church, [whose parishioners think] they're getting a male minister. Pasture is the family's last name, and she's a little green, being a new [parent], being a new minister, being in a new town. It's a very family thing. PAX is looking at it. There are several other things, too, but that one right now is the hot one.

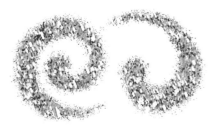

SHOOTING STARS

Over the years, I've been lucky enough to work with some of daytime television's biggest stars—true leaders among leading ladies. But you don't want to hear about that from lil' ol' me. Instead, since a picture says a thousand words, let's let this portfolio of women with whom I've worked speak the volumes about them that I couldn't possibly.

KELLY RIPA

Since leaving her *All My Children* role of plucky Hayley Santos, this ambitious blonde has gone on to headline her own sitcom, *Hope & Faith*, and give Regis Philbin more perk than a double latte as co-host of *Live with Regis and Kelly*.

Photo by Robert Milazzo

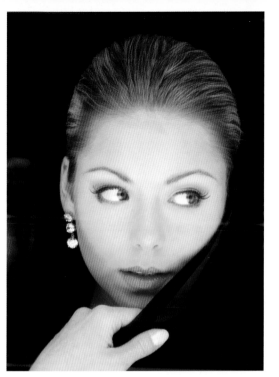

JORDANA BREWSTER

Following her stint as naughty Nikki Munson on *As the World Turns*, this rising star made tracks for the big screen, joining another ex-daytimer, Paul Walker, in *The Fast and the Furious*. She'll next be seen opposite James Franco in the film *Annapolis*.

Photo by Greg Weiner
Photo Courtesy of Soaps in Depth

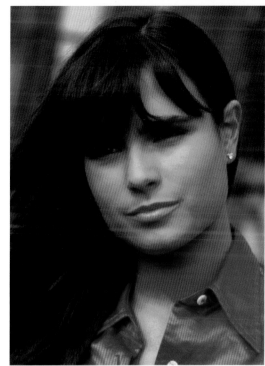

TAMMY BLANCHARD

Shortly after leaving behind *Guiding Light* and Drew Jacobs, the conflicted character she'd created, this up-and-comer won an Emmy for the TV movie *Life with Judy Garland: Me and My Shadows* and was a Tony nominee for *Gypsy*.

Photo by Greg Weiner
Photo Courtesy of Soaps in Depth

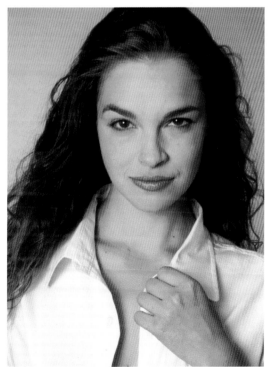

SYDNEY PENNY

Since making herself at home in daytime television, the child star of TV's *The Thorn Birds* has been dubbed a queen of drama, thanks to her knack for playing tortured heroines (currently The *Bold & the Beautiful*'s Samantha Kelly).

Photo by Robert Milazzo

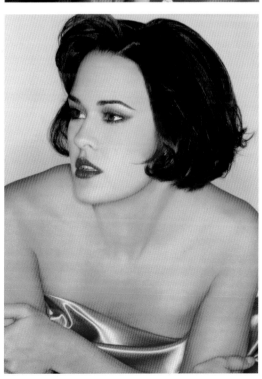

KIM ZIMMER

This Emmy winner has done more soaps than the Zest company. But it is as *Guiding Light*'s scarlet woman, Reva Lewis, that she will always be most vividly remembered.

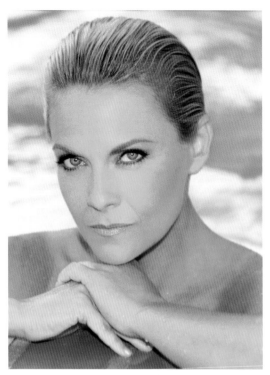

CYNTHIA WATROS

Still basking in the afterglow of her Emmy victory—for her stunning depiction of *Guiding Light* nurse Annie Dutton's descent into madness—this born comedienne landed one sitcom (*The Drew Carey Show*) after another (*Titus*). She'll next be seen in the feature *American Crude*, with *Scrubs*' John C. McGinley.

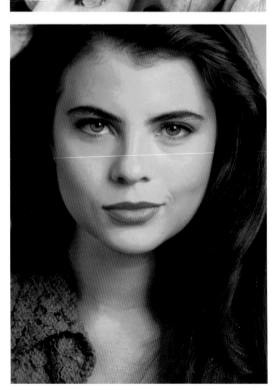

SARAH MICHELLE GELLAR

An Emmy in hand for her performance as conniving Kendall Hart on *All My Children*, this future icon went and scored the role of a lifetime: the lead in the cult phenomenon *Buffy the Vampire Slayer*. Since then, she's become a multiplex mainstay and even brought home a matinee idol of her own—hubby Freddie Prinze Jr.

WENDY MONIZ

Once she was done wreaking havoc as *Guiding Light*'s demented Dinah Marler, this standout went Hollywood— and quickly was signed to be a series regular on the legal drama *The Guardian*.

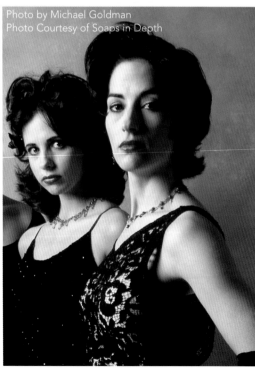

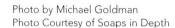

YASMINE BLEETH

Once she'd earned her soap stripes as *Ryan's Hope* sweetheart Ryan Fenelli and *One Life to Live* sweet-tart Lee Ann Buchanan, this *Baywatch* babe began making TV movies, seemingly at a rate of one a day.

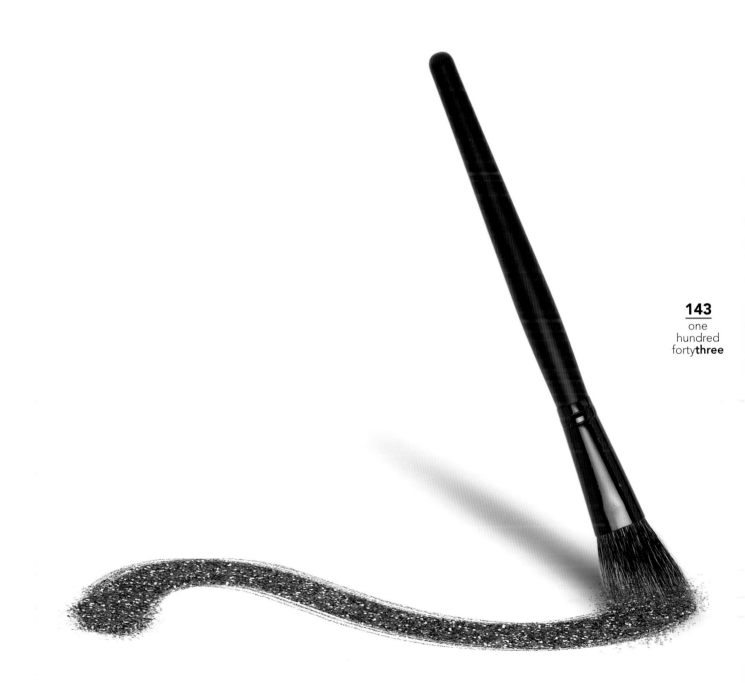

POSTSCRIPT:

Attitude Adjustment

Th-th-that's all, folks. Stick a fork in it; this book is done. Don't you feel prettier?

Seriously, now that you have read all my advice (and gone off with me on my tangents—which, history tells us, are where the most interesting things in life are always found), I *do* hope you are feeling prettier—or at least less intimidated by your make-up bag. (If you're going to be intimidated by a bag, let it be a Kate Spade, and, by all means, let the price tag be the scary part.) I also hope you will remember that this, like any beauty book, is just one individual's (admittedly learned) views on make-up. It will be of no use whatsoever to you until you apply the fundamental strategies and techniques I've discussed to your own face (and life). *That's* when the magic happens!

Lastly, and most importantly—I hope that you have begun to think about your looks as something that goes beyond skin-deep. If you have, good—because the way you feel about how you look can and does make all the difference in how you actually *do* look. By extension, if you feel that you look good, you will feel better in general, which can only help you look better, too. (For you smartasses reading this, no, that is not a chicken-and-the-egg conundrum: First comes feeling good, then looking good, and so forth. It's like a wheel that doesn't begin to turn until you feel good. So there!)

The tricky part about what should actually be so simple—accept and embrace the way you look, and other people will, too—is that we are strangely willing, even eager, to let others influence our opinion of ourselves. Why do we do it? Are they around when we wake up at the crack of dawn with eye boogers and bedhead? Have they seen the way we've struggled to lose that two and a half pounds for the fourth time? Heck, no. So why would we give them this power that they don't deserve? They're about as qualified to judge our looks as Paula Abdul is to critique an *American Idol* performance. Even worse, this submission to rampant criticism leads many girls that I meet to harbor self-esteem that's so low, they treat themselves horribly—and often allow others to do so as well. (I'm not sure which is more appalling.) So if nothing else, if all you needed was a little confidence, I hope this book has given you a big, heaping dose.

Now then, if what you need to feel good about yourself and your looks goes *beyond* confidence, then please—even though I just told you to pooh-pooh the things that folks may say to you—listen to *me* when I say, "Get some help. Do the work. Take the plunge." Nobody can make you feel better but you. This means that you have to initiate the change and carry it through—and it's tough. But it's worth it. Actually, that's one of my mantras (yes, another one): You're worth it. If you're sitting there thinking, "I dunno. Am I, really?" then you really need a reality check. You *are*. I am. We all are.

I know of whence I speak, too: My self-esteem tends to be so low that I sometimes trip over it. But I'm working on it, and I'll keep working on it until I've got it licked. And here's the good news: Learning to be kind to yourself doesn't involve only the kind of histrionics you see on *Dr. Phil*. I try to elevate my opinion of myself by flat-out improving myself—and kiddies, that is *fun*! I've gone back to school, I get massages and pedicures, I've joined a gym, and, best of all, I take time every day just for me. This says to me, and I guess now to all of you, "Hey, I'm important. I deserve a moment. And by God, I'm going to take one!"

I happen to know that a number of the actresses in this book subscribe to that same theory of self-preservation: making time for yourself so you can make the most of your time.

Wait. Wait. Stop everything. Are you saying to yourself, "Yeah, but hello?! They're soap stars. I'm just a lowly [insert your occupation here]."

Well, I can't argue with you about the soap star part—they *are* soap stars. But they are also wives and moms, business-people and baseball coaches. In other words, they're just women, busy, resourceful and strong, just like you. That's why, even as you've looked at their pictures and read their stories, the focus of this book has remained squarely on you—you are them, they are you. This book wasn't designed as a pedestal from which they could brag; it was created as a forum through which I hoped you could relate.

In fact, the next time you turn on one of their shows, I hope you watch these women with a new perspective. They are brilliant actresses, one and all, certainly. But you are on a level playing field with every one of them. In your own way, in your own right, *you* are a star. I know that sounds so corny, you're probably thinking that Richard Simmons wrote this chapter. But it's true. If you can't accept that at first, then think about the important women in your life. Maybe it's your mom or a friend or your sister. For me, God bless her, it's my Aunt Kathy. Do you think

I feel that Robin Mattson or Fiona Hutchison is cooler than my Aunt Kathy? No way! They're cool, sure. But not cooler. Once you can see that these actresses are no different or better than the real-life women you respect, perhaps you will find it easier to acknowledge that they're also no cooler, or lovelier, than you. More than 100 pages later, you ought to know that I'm telling you the truth. Now, all you have to do is, ahem, face it.

"accept and embrace the way you look"

These days, every time you turn on the TV, Corporate America is getting a bum rap—and maybe some firms deserve it. But I have to say, as I was putting this book together for Gilda's Club, a number of companies bent over backwards to make the experience truly (bear with me) beautiful. So, for their help and generosity—and for always supplying me with toys I can take to my own personal playground—I gratefully acknowledge the following companies:

M A C

K E V Y N   A U C O I N   B E A U T Y

freeze 24·7™

girlactik BEAUTY

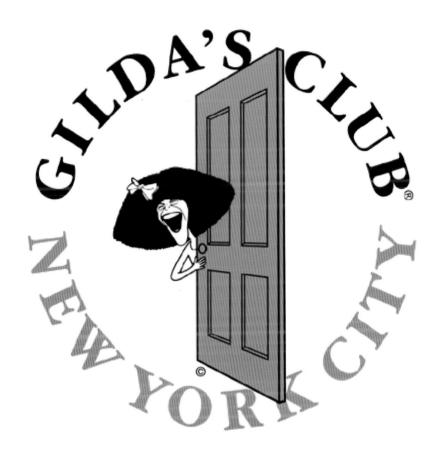

Living with cancer?
Come as you are.™

A percentage of the proceeds will benefit Gilda's Club.

GILDA'S CLUB   195 WEST HOUSTON STREET, NYC, NY 10014   212.647.9700